Talking Medicine

W · W · NORTON & COMPANY · NEW YORK · LONDON

Talking Medicine

America's Doctors Tell Their Stories

Peter MacGarr Rabinowitz

Library of Congress Cataloging in Publication Data
Rabinowitz, Peter MacGarr.
Talking medicine.

1. Physicians—United States—Interviews. I. Title.
[DNLM: 1. Medicine—United States—Personal
narratives.   2. Physicians—United States—Personal narratives. WZ140 AA1 R115]
R153.R32   1981   610.69'52'0973   80–18553
ISBN 0–393–01397–9

W. W. Norton & Company, Inc. 500 Fifth Avenue, New York, N.Y. 10110
W. W. Norton & Company Ltd. 25 New Street Square, London EC4A 3NT

1 2 3 4 5 6 7 8 9 0

FOR ALAN AND DOTTIE

Contents

*Pseudonym

*Pseudonym

Preface

This book documents a personal search to discover what it is like to be a doctor in America today. The search began two years ago when I found myself, like many of my college classmates, wondering whether to embark on a medical career. Like most of them, I had little direct knowledge of the American medical profession.

"I wanted to be a doctor," wrote Albert Schweitzer, "that I might be able to work without having to talk." And since the time of Asclepius, the medical profession has wrapped a cloud of secrecy about its inner workings.

But how was I to know whether I wanted to be a doctor, if I could not penetrate that cloud? Days spent roaming through large libraries produced no book that permitted me to answer this question. There were biographies of medical demigods such as Osler, Harvey, and Lister that only obscured the picture with hero worship. There were autobiographies by several physicians who had found time to write; but these were solitary voices, and there were not many. And finally there were many books written about America's "health-care crisis" by everyone from economists to philosophers. These tended to attack the medical profession with enough virulence to make them as unbelievable as the fawning biographies of medical greats.

So I decided to talk to doctors myself. I wanted to hear their side of the story.

At first my goal lay in an uncharted wilderness, since I knew personally only five or six of the nation's 400,000 physicians. But my desire to know more about medicine increased steadily as the decision of whether to go to medical school became imminent.

The doctors I knew introduced me to ten or fifteen more, and my project gained momentum. "You've got to talk to Dr. Blank," one physician would advise me. "He [or she] will tell you a story you'll never forget."

Yet some of the doctors I requested interviews with were initially resistant. Who was I, and exactly how did I plan to use these interviews? Sometimes a secretary would politely inform me that the doctor was simply too busy for many months to come.

Several months after I first had the idea to talk with doctors, I was accepted into medical school. I had discovered the peculiar, almost irresistible fascination of medicine. And I decided to write a book about my conversations with doctors.

"You're one of us now; you're on the inside," said a cardiac surgeon, offering me a cigarette. I had no further difficulty arranging interviews. Almost every doctor was eager to tell a beginning medical student "what medicine is all about, since most premedical and medical students don't realize what they're getting themselves into."

This book is a compilation of what the doctors I spoke with felt that I was getting myself into. And woven through their words of advice and perspective are threads of intensely personal experiences.

They met with me in their book-lined offices; in clattering hospital cafeterias; amid the white-coated bustle of hospital wards; in the electrified atmosphere of operating rooms; in the quiet of their homes. Often I felt I was witnessing that rare moment in a person's life when the whirl of activity ceases, if only for a few hours. At such a time the mind has a chance to wander over the events, emotions, and reasonings that led to the present. I found most of the doctors to be open and sometimes almost desperately eager to share confidences and opinions that had few other outlets. Many of the physicians and medical students whom I interviewed appear here under assumed names, in the interest of their professional protection. Some requested this expressly, making it clear that their feelings and insights must not become known to their patients or even to their colleagues.

After two years, during which I traveled around the United States interviewing more than seventy physicians, I assembled the twenty-four interviews that I felt would be as informative and interesting to a reader as the actual conversations had been for me. I wanted to write the book that I had been looking for in those libraries two years before, a book whose primary purpose would be closing the gap in communication between doctors and the public.

While editing thousands of pages of interview transcript, I came to see that I was dealing with a language slightly different from normal English. This "medicalese" is an odd alloy of colloquial English, science-textbook prose, and abbreviated jargon that is the accepted means of communication on the wards. This dialect can be euphemistic; "fever of unknown origin" (i.e., no one knows what is going on) can be dignified as "idiopathic hyperthermia," or shortened to "F.U.O." In this way, "medicalese" becomes convoluted and unintelligible to nonmedical readers and listeners.

It was necessary to translate the interviews into something closer to spoken English. I have tried hard, however, to retain unique tones of each physician's voice, for this is a book about people.

In arranging the interviews into their present form, I have felt like an apprentice working in mosaics, choosing the colorful, asymmetric tiles that together will form a coherent portrait. In this case it is the portrait of a profession. Such a mosaic requires glue and backing, and I have provided relevant background information and introductions to each interview.

"When I was in medical school," many of the doctors would begin. And it is along the vertical lines of a medical career that I have structured this book. The early sections parallel how the years of education lead inexorably to residencies and later practice or research. The later sections of the book portray some physicians looking inward, evaluating personal lives, and others stepping back to take a longer look at their lives, at the "big picture."

Two years after beginning both medical school and the writing of this book, I cannot claim that doctors are very different from anyone else. Like most people they feel an urge for security, for achievement, for understanding. Like most people they wish to help others to cope with human frailty and death. But in no other group of people have I seen these simple desires and ideals so richly fulfilled and also so severely tested, even overwhelmed. In these stories of physicians' lives, these basic human drives are often glaringly obvious, stripped of mystery. It is possible to see which hopes are real, which ones are impossible of realization, which ones are merely platitudes. What happens depends on the individual physician.

There is a widespread belief that the rigors of medical school and residency training change idealistic students into hardened professionals. Medical education and training, according to this belief, somehow condition doctors to act in a certain way. But I believe that the most critical factor is the nature of the people who decide to go to medical school, not what is done to them later.

After residency training, doctors have an unusual amount of freedom. As one doctor confided to me, "Medicine is the only profession where one can still be an entrepreneur." Doctors practice under remarkably few governmental regulations or economic constraints. Even given the specter of malpractice suits, medical practice remains one of the most flexible and profitable of occupations.

Considering this degree of freedom, why should the rates of suicide, drug addiction, and alcoholism be so high among physicians? Why do recent opinion polls show public confidence in physicians to be at a new low? Why should the same polls show that a majority of Americans believe there is a "health-care crisis" in this country? And why are there at this writing several bills before Congress that call for major revisions in America's health-care system?

It must have something to do with the kind of people who have become doctors in the past. I began writing this book wondering, Who are the doctors of America? As I listened to their stories, I started to ask, Who should be doctors in the future?

The fate of medicine lies in the hands of those people now making up their minds whether to go to medical school. This book is written for them, and for everyone interested in looking behind the stereotyped image of the physician. Its purpose is to inform, to warn, and to encourage—and, perhaps in the process, to entertain.

Introduction

ROBERT COLES

There are many ways a particular profession can be regarded. American medicine, for instance, has been closely scrutinized in recent years by social historians, demographers, political scientists, and public-policy analysts, not to mention the wonderfully wise and eloquent essayist Lewis Thomas. Novelists have also traditionally been interested in doctors. Through characters such as George Eliot's Lydgate, or Sinclair Lewis's Martin Arrowsmith, and, most recently, Dr. Walker Percy's interesting and exceedingly perplexed Dr. Sutter and Dr. More, readers have had a chance to examine the ironies, ambiguities, paradoxes, inconsistencies, and contradictions that plague all human life—true—but take a special form in one or another kind of life, certainly including that of the doctor. The novel, of course, is especially suited to examine moral textures—the ways in which we try to uphold professed ideals, or the manner in which we make subtle or not so subtle compromises, if not outright betrayals, of principle. Novelists, too, bring us as close as we are likely to get, short of direct observation, to the actual rhythms of a given kind of human experience—those sights and sounds, those exchanges of opinion and sentiment, that characterize one rather than another aspect of everyday life. Most of us, however, don't stop to give our personal stories the form a novel requires. We are not, that is, inclined to use our imaginations systematically, in such a way that "life" and "art" become not polarities but elements in a writer's struggle to comprehend this world—our hopes and worries, our aspirations and limitations, our conceits and deceits, our victories and losses.

In recent years a field called "oral history" has commanded a good deal of attention, and deservedly so when it has been practiced by the likes of Oscar Lewis, Theodore Rosengarten, and Studs Terkel, all sensitive listeners, astute observers, and, not least, shrewd narrators, who are aware that the documentary tradition, no less than that of fiction, requires coherence, structure, and a sifting and sorting that nourishes detail, respects complexity, illuminates whatever symmetry has been found, and, very important, helps us get to the heart of a given matter—a life's essential features. As is always so, it seems, a "new" field can become an occasion for extravagant claims or mean-spirited objections. Too often we end up overlooking historical continuities—as if, for example, ancient Greece had not more than a passing acquaintance with "oral history." Still, that expression provides an umbrella for some significant and original social research now going on—work done not with "material" or "data" or statistics, but with men and women and children, often enough so-called "ordinary" human beings (who, of course, turn out to be, on close observation, extraordinary). To such a literature this book surely belongs, as a strong, energetic, wide-ranging addition. A medical student has roamed a big nation and come up with a varied cast of characters, so to speak, each of whom offers us a singular means of entry into the medical profession. The result is a compelling mix of fact and subjectivity, and, for the reader, an education about "how it goes" in one segment of a nation's professional life.

These are stories, unashamedly collected, edited, and finally connected, by a thoughtful and knowing young man who has taken the time to approach (and win over) all sorts of future colleagues: struggling students and apprentices, unknown and unheralded, but sometimes utterly high-minded and generous doctors, who work in small towns or in the neighborhoods of our cities; big shots who run institutions, laboratories, professional organizations—a virtual rainbow of individuals, united only, it seems, by membership in a profession the knowledge of which means very much to each and every one of us. A portrait of that profession is, it can be said, delivered to us "in the round" through the autobiographical statements that follow—a display of the high ideals, the decent and kind moments, and also the warts and worse, which are devastatingly conveyed in the words of certain men and women whose smugness or self-satisfaction or callousness or financial and careerist aggrandizement are obvious. There is to be found in these pages, also, a lot of good-will, sensitivity, and ethical passion—many reminders that Christ's remonstrance "Physician, heal thyself" does not go altogether un-heeded by those American men and women who have chosen to enter and remain within one of the most demanding of occupations. And that a promising, morally discerning medical student such as the author of this book has been able to embark upon and complete so successfully his inquiry tells us something, too—about the open-ness, the candid responsiveness, and the intense self-scrutiny that characterize a good deal of medical life in America today.

ACKNOWLEDGMENTS

This book would not have come about without the generosity of the many physicians and medical students who shared their stories with me. Many of the interviews I conducted do not appear here, but the perspectives gleaned from each and every discussion have enriched the process of preparing this book.

Special thanks to Charles Bodemer, Zenaido Camacho, Janet Finnie, Naomi Pascal, and Brian Wilson, who gave encouragement and guidance while the book was still in embryonic stages.

My typist, Andrea Valesko, somehow deciphered hundreds of hours of cassette tapes made under highly varied circumstances. Her neat transcripts were invaluable in turning the interviews into a readable form.

The following are a few of the people who offered suggestions and assistance along the way: Margaret Anderson, Josh Benditt, Tom Chase, Tom Crawford, Jackie Dalecki, Joan Feeney, Durlin Hickock, Susan Jackson, Mary Kamb, Joyce McKenney, Andrew Rutten, Jon Sheffer, and John Sundsten.

My family offered constant support, and my grandmother, Anna Wolf, proved to be my most demanding editor.

PART I

Education

. . . From the standpoint of the young student, the school is, of course, concerned chiefly with his acquisition of the proper knowledge, attitude, and technique. Once more, it matters not at that stage whether his destination is to be investigation or practice. In either case, as beginner, he learns chiefly what is old, known, understood. But the old, known, and understood are all alike new to him. . . .

—Abraham Flexner, *Medical Education in the United States and Canada*, 1910

Among certain "primitive" societies, an occasional young man would begin acting strangely around the time of puberty. He would let out wild shouts in public for no particular reason, tear at his hair, climb up and down trees in a frenzy of senseless activity. After proving his aberrancy beyond a shadow of a doubt, the youth would disappear, alone, into the wilderness. Some time later he would reappear, subdued and possessing a calm sense of direction about the course his life should take. His old friends, even his family, now treated him with respect mixed with fear, keeping their distance. For such a youth was now ready to begin his formal training to be a shaman—a tribal healer.

If there is a modern-day counterpart for this "preshamanistic psychosis," as anthropologists call it, it is the years of pre-med and medical education.

Strange, solemn institutions—the medical schools of this country. Clustered in urban areas, these conglomerates of lecture hall, laboratory, and hospital go about their business of granting 16,000 M.D. degrees every year.

Following Abraham Flexner's report to the Carnegie Commission in 1910, the miscellaneous nineteenth-century medical schools—often no more than one-year diploma mills—gave way to a handful of demanding, expensive, standardized centers for learning and research. Their suddenly uniform curriculum synthesized German methods of basic-science instruction and the British "clerking" system of clinical experience. For a period generally lasting four years, a medical student meshes with faculty, administrators, and other health professionals. There is a coherence, a seductiveness about the process that is so great that only one student in one hundred fails to graduate.

And yet—a professor of neurology wrinkled his brow and gazed out the window of his medical school office. "It's eerie," he mused, "to see students arrive all full of ideas and freshness, and then each year become progressively homogenous, as if to fit some unseen mold. Is it something we do to them, something they do to themselves?"

A fourth-year student gave a cynical laugh as he told about serving on his school's admissions committee. All twenty-six applicants he interviewed insisted that they were different from the pre-med crowd—that they would never change to become callous, selfish, and conservative like the doctors they had known. When the student asked each applicant why not, "The same damn answer came back every time: because they were aware of the pitfalls, because they would stay on top of things and not let med school get to them. And you know, that's exactly what I said, four years ago. . . ."

Getting In

"The privileges of the medical school," Flexner wrote, "can no longer be open to casual strollers from the highway. It is necessary to install a doorkeeper who will, by careful scrutiny, ascertain the fitness of the applicant."

In 1977, more than 40,000 premedical students applied to the 119 medical schools across the country. Of the 16,000 who gained entrance, more than half had been "A" students in college. Most of them were caucasian men from upper-middle-class backgrounds, and one in ten was the child of a physician.

It was February, and Tim Morton had been in medical school for five months. He had successfully passed his first round of exams and laughed when I asked him to talk about getting into medical school.

"Do I have to go back over all that misery?" he asked, sitting down at the snack bar in the basement of the medical-school complex. It was evening, and the room was deserted except for the janitor scrubbing floors and three students preparing for an exam at another table. Slight of build and wearing a Hawaiian shirt, Tim stroked his full, dark beard and focused playful eyes on his cup of coffee.

"Oh, well," he said, "here goes. . . ."

When I first decided that I wanted to do this, I was a sophomore in high school. I come from a goal-oriented family, and my parents said I had to decide what I was going to do. So I started looking around: my older brother is a lawyer, and I watched him and decided that I didn't have a logical mind and that anyway I had a distaste for the law. My dad was a salesman and had been a carpenter before, and none of that appealed to me. Business didn't appeal to me, because I have a distaste for money too.

At the time, I was playing violin and my teacher was very overbearing, and she had decided for me that I was going to be a professional musician. I started thinking about it and looking at her and her life and the musicians I'd known, and decided that professional musicians are a very unhappy, narrow-minded bunch of people with closed lives. So it was kind of hard telling my teacher that I was changing her plans, but I had to.

You know, I was feeling lost. I didn't want to be a teacher, because I never had much respect for the teachers that taught me. And the only other thing I was doing at the time was commercial art, so I looked at that very carefully and finally decided that I didn't have any talent.

Then my parents read in the newspaper about a symposium at the university on medical careers, and so for three days in the summer I took the bus out from Issaquah to the university and stayed at the symposium for eight hours a day. There were people from all the different programs: nursing, physical therapy, all the specialties of medicine, and I was just fascinated. I couldn't believe how interesting it sounded, and I decided right then to study medicine.

I started to find out what you had to do to get into med school; I found out about pre-med and asked a lot of questions about where I should go to college. The one school I could afford was Bellevue Community College, and they told me that they had a .001 percent acceptance rate into medical school, so I started looking for other ways to put myself through college. My brother had gone to Princeton on a full scholarship, so I applied there, and he suggested that I apply to Harvard. I thought Harvard was in New York, and I didn't want to go to New York, but I applied anyway, and when I found out it was in Boston that was a big relief, and they accepted me and gave me a scholarship.

When I got to Harvard, the first thing I did was disguise the fact that I was pre-med, 'cause I'd heard all these terrible rumors about how you're socially ostracized if people know you're pre-med. I had spoken to a man who once had been on the admissions committee at the University of Washington Medical School, and I'd asked him what to study in college. He'd said that admissions committees love the "renaissance man," a person that can do science and music and art and philosophy and sports, the whole bit, and he'd asked me what I was interested in. I'd told him I wasn't sure, but I'd read maybe three novels in my life, and English sounded like a neat field. He said, "Well, do that, that's wonderful, we just love English majors." He said, "Just take your pre-med requirements and then take anything else you want." So I trotted off to college with this misconception and became an English major—composition and poetry, Shakespeare and James Joyce, and all sorts of short stories. In the meantime I was taking pre-med courses, and with my terrible math and science background I couldn't understand the calculus, and the chemistry I was taking required calculus. It was terrible; I was floundering in everything I did; I just wished I could die. But I had one roommate who was very nice and was a physics major and knew all the math and chemistry, and he helped me along. By the second year, I felt I had caught up with everyone else. I took one year of inorganic chemistry, one year of organic, one year of physics, one year of biology, and one year of calculus. During my junior year I finally let someone in on the fact that I wanted to be a doctor—I talked to the pre-med adviser in my dorm. She looked at my record and looked at what I was doing and then told me bluntly that I would never get in anywhere, period, that it was a very expensive process to apply, and that I shouldn't bother. I guess she was looking especially at my freshman grades, which were C's and C+'s, which I didn't think were *that* bad—I was happy to have survived. I figured that this adviser was considering the types of medical schools that Harvard students usually apply to—Duke and Yale and Harvard and Stanford. Since all I wanted was to go to the University of Washington, which is a state school, I decided to ignore her, which was foolish; it's difficult to get into *any* medical school.

One thing I did during my college summers to see if I really wanted to be a doctor was to work as an orderly in a hospital. I emptied bed pans and helped put in catheters and worked in the morgue, and learned more about medicine than in anything else I had done, because I was kind of invisible. I was this strange-looking little kid in a white uniform—everyone thought I was about fifteen. I would be working on a patient and the doctor would walk in. I would step away and the doctor would pretend I wasn't there, as if to say, "This guy doesn't have the brains to understand what I am saying, so I can say anything I want to." I got to observe good doctors and bad doctors and mediocre doctors and cruel doctors. I made sure I was in the right place at the right time—if they wanted to do a spinal tap they'd look around and here was this male body standing in the corner, and they'd say, "Hey you, get over here." And I'd go over and kneel on the bed and hold the patient by the neck and the knees—hold them still so the doctor could do the puncture. I would watch the doctor and how he was treating the patient, and I began to have strong feelings that many patients were mistreated, but I was powerless to do much about it. Anyone who is going to be a doctor should spend some time being that low on the totem pole.

At the end of my junior year, I sent my applications in to twelve medical schools and got fucked over by AMCAS, the central application service, which put my application in the wrong box, then found it ten days after the deadline and sent me a nasty note saying that if 30,000 other students could get things in on time it was amazing that I couldn't.

Finally I got interviewed by the University of Washington, by Pittsburgh, and by Cincinnati. The University of Washington interview was the worst. I was late for it because it was Christmas vacation and I had to fly in. There was a snowstorm in Boston, and I slept in the Boston airport for two nights and then got to Chicago, where I had to spend another night in the airport. I arrived in Seattle at twelve noon, and my interview was at 12:30. My mother met me at the airport. She had brought a pair of scissors in her purse in case I had let my hair grow too long, and she brought along a sports coat and tie and a shirt, all of which belonged to my older brother, who is at least six inches taller than I am. I walked into the interview with the sports coat hanging over my knuckles, and my tie was tied all wrong since I had hardly ever worn one, and I was in a daze from three nights in airports.

I was surprised by the questions they asked me. They weren't interested in why I wanted to be a doctor. Instead, they asked very pointed questions about why my freshman year at college had gone so poorly. I explained that I thought I had been poorly prepared. The man said, "Well, what makes you think you're not poorly prepared for medical school?" I said, "You know, I've been kicked around a lot in college and I don't think it could possibly happen again—I'm not that green." Then they started asking me questions about why I was an English major. I said, "Well, I wanted to have a well-rounded education and wanted to be a 'renaissance man,' I mean, there would not be time during medical school to read *Hamlet* in depth." They said, "Yes, but why were you an English major?" I asked, "Do you mean as opposed to being a history major?" "No," they said, why hadn't I majored in the sciences? I told them the advice I had been given before I started college, and they said, "Oh well, we did consider that to be appropriate at one time, but now 85 percent of each class are chemistry and biology majors." There had been a change in strategy, since the well-rounded people flunked too many med-school courses. Looking back on it, it makes sense, since the school is interested in putting out a product at the least possible cost, which means having a low attrition rate. So they had developed a distaste for Ivy League humanities majors.

Anyway, I did my interviews and came back to school, and the mountain of rejection letters began to form. I took thumbtacks and stuck the letters to the ceiling above my desk. Soon it was covered with paper. "Dear Reject, Sorry you're so stupid. Yours sincerely. . . ." The last rejection I got was from the University of Washington.

When I graduated I had a degree in English and was unemployable. I got a job emptying garbage cans at Lake Sammamish State Park, until one of my mother's friends who is a professor found out what I was doing and became incensed. She asked around until she found a research assistantship that was opening up—working in cardiac pathology. When I first went in and talked with the doctor about the job, I just about gagged—I'm sort of squeamish—and he told me I would be doing autopsies and perfusing the coronary arteries of hearts with gelatin, and dissecting the hearts and x-raying the vessels. It was hard at first. I had no research experience, but I ended up working with the project for two years, and medicine became more important to me because I could see directly what medicine could do for bodies. Working so much around dead people, I lost my belief that there could be a soul which flies off into the air or sinks into the ground when someone dies. For me there could be no distinction between body and mind, no separation between spirit and the machinery of the physical self. When the body stops functioning, that personality which goes along with it also ceases to function, and that's the end of it. I became much more careful with the bodies than did some of my co-workers who felt that some sort of soul had left, that a corpse was a house which was no longer being used. I felt it was still a person, even though the machinery for feeling pain or recognizing the indignities of an autopsy had stopped functioning at death. The human body and the spirit or personality or soul had become for me inseparable. While that may be a sad philosophy to have come up with, it reaffirmed my desire to get into med school.

I went to the woman who had found me the job and asked her for help. She looked over my record and explained to me that most of getting into med school was politics, in the sense that you have to present yourself in the most favorable light and appear to be the sort of person that the medical school is looking for. I waited a year and a half to apply again, and during that time I did the research project and took courses during my lunch hour—courses that she helped me select and which had impressive titles—genetics, microbiology, biochemistry. She said whatever you do, make sure that you get the top grade in your class, and see that the teacher mentions that you got the top grade in your class. So I went about deliberately getting the top grades, and it was odd for me because I had never worked for grades, but I took very selected courses and got very good grades, and got letters of recommendation from the two doctors I was working with and from this woman, and then I reapplied. I called up the financial-aid office of Harvard and got the names of all the scholarship awards I had been given so that I could list all these important names as "honors," when actually they were just the names of scholarships. I had a long list of the things I had done in college—plays I had been in, commercial art I had done, orchestras I had played in. I asked different people for advice on this and was told "Well, they don't give a shit about this, but this looks good, but don't mention this," and so on. I wrote my personal statement after talking with four different people about it, and when it was done each sentence was perfect and it filled the space on the application exactly, and it consisted of very factual summaries of where I went to high school, where I went to college, the awards I had won, you know, Merit Scholar and all that stuff. I wrote a little paragraph about my research, in which I used as many large words as possible, making sure that they were all accurate. After that I talked for a brief sentence about why I wanted to be a doctor. I offered no opinions at all, I just stated that I thought being a doctor was good, whereas my past application had been this frothing, foaming essay on the doctor's position in society and how patients ought to be treated. The woman who was advising me had warned me not to have any opinions. She said that med schools aren't interested in green-horn idealistic people who want to change the system—they want people who understand that the system is there because it is the best possible system. Playing this political game made me feel morally bankrupt, but I wanted to be a doctor badly enough to play the game.

I made sure that my application was mailed the very first day, mailed to arrive at AMCAS the very day that their offices opened. I kept very careful records of everything that I sent off, and when I took the MCATs over again I took out all my old textbooks and for two months before the test I'd sit in bed every night and read a few chapters, and did all the practice problems. I still didn't do as well as I wanted, but I was very consistent.

The second interview was completely different. They didn't ask me anything about my past academic records. Before I went in, a bunch of my friends who were first-year medical students got together and collected all of the questions they'd been asked in their interviews, and we all got together in the pizza parlor and they asked me questions. So when my interview started, they asked me a question about world health which I'd prepared for, so I sat there for a few seconds to try and look as if this was a totally new question, and then I rattled off this amazing answer. They started asking me more and more pointed questions which began to evolve into moralistic issues—euthanasia, sterilization, abortion, legal and religious problems of blood transfusion, that sort of thing. One man on the board was getting more and more antsy, because every answer I was coming up with was full of facts and statistics and current theories, and no opinions—I was careful not to have any opinions. Finally he said, "Well, why do you want to be a doctor?" I had a very pat answer about the need for doctors in this country, and he said, "Yes, but why do *you* want to be a doctor?" He said he knew what I was doing by witholding my opinions, and he finally said, "What is your opinion *personally*, why do you, personally, want to be a doctor?" I looked at him for a few seconds and said, "Do you really want to know?" He said yes, and I told him, "I want to do something worthwhile with my life. I don't want to fritter it away, and of all the things I've looked at medicine seems to be the most likely avenue for my being useful. And I want to be a doctor because it will be interesting and I'll learn about my own body, I'll be able to help other people; but actually it's selfish—I want to be useful." The man sat back and sighed, and I could see it relieved him to find that I had finally offered an opinion. After that they let me go. Even though I felt that the second interview went worse than the first, I got in a month after the second interview, which was a great relief.

First Year

Dr. Julius Kaas, Professor of Anatomy

Dr. Julius Kaas, M.D., Ph.D., stood, bony arms akimbo, in front of the first-year medical-school class. Although his upper spine hunched forward slightly, he was tall and athletically lean under a tight-fitting cotton jersey and European slacks. Short-cropped curls were drawn back from his high forehead, and his narrow face ended in a perfectly trimmed Mephistophelian beard.

"I want to introduce you to Human Biology 511: anatomy and embryology of the human thorax and abdomen." His foreign accent impatiently cut off consonants and stretched vowels to the breaking point: "ahnaaahtomy." His large green eyes searched the rows of restless, worried faces. Although it was only the end of orientation week, Dr. Kaas had memorized every student's face and name from the class composite picture.

"Now, many physicians will tell you that anatomy is not an important part of a medical education, that you will soon forget it. Yet I submit to you, and you must remember this, that when you become clinicians and you examine human bodies every day, the thought process you will go through will utilize the anatomy that I am going to present in this course. Before you can understand diseased bodies, you must learn to see and appreciate normality."

From the middle of the classroom came the sound of someone suddenly writhing, striking a desk, then sliding to the floor. A student's arm quivered, then disappeared from view, and two doctors who had just given a lecture on humanistic medicine walked brusquely along the row to kneel beside the collapsed student. They raised him up unconscious and carried him into the hall. There was a minute of excited conversation in the room, and then Dr. Kaas, who had not moved, spoke again.

"I think we can resume now, class, but I feel you have heard enough introduction for the time being. Let us go upstairs and meet the cadavers."

Minutes later, Dr. Kaas addressed the students who were grouped in fours around each of the twenty-five dissecting tables. On every table was a long, white-shrouded mound. The laboratory air was heavy with formaldehyde fumes.

"I want you to remember, class, that you are very privileged to be able to work with human specimens. Each person willed his or her body to the department of biological structure, it was a matter of free choice. Accordingly, I would like you to give each cadaver all the respect that is due a living person. Now, please draw back the top sheet." There was the sound of plastic being turned back on itself. "Very good," Kaas intoned, "and now, please remove the second sheet."

There was a hiss of sodden cloth lifting off a wet surface. Then the room was very silent for a few seconds.

The autumn quarter continued in this way. Three days into the term, students took scalpels and sliced their cadavers' chests from throat to umbilical. Kaas moved from table to table, greeting students by name and urging, "This is the longest cut you will ever make, even if you become a surgeon, so I want you to be bold and enjoy it."

In lectures he exhorted the class to follow him more closely: "It is not enough for you to know where a structure is and what embryonic layer it is derived from and what its Latin name is. I want you to be able to really see it. Today, I want you to be little fairies, standing on the lesser curvature of the stomach. If you walk anteriorly, you will have to descend to the surface of the greater omentum. If you walk posteriorly, you will come to the wall of the lesser sac; and if you follow this medially, you will come to the epiploic foramen. It's really very simple [groans from the class], but you must sit your butt in a chair and work at it until you can draw all of this by heart. Don't look at the book each time. I assure you, the book has it right. You must get it right in your own head; come and see me if you are having trouble. Everything has been going quite well so far, but you must keep preparing for every lecture, you must keep up with the material, or you will be completely lost by the time we enter the perineum. Now, let me draw this for you one more time." His long fingers would reach for a new color of chalk, and soon more sweeping and complex patterns would appear on the blackboard.

The professors of the other courses—biochemistry, physiology, histology, interviewing skills—complained frequently that students were spending almost all their time studying anatomy. Yet the course only accelerated. Half the class failed the midterm, and Kaas became relentless, irritable. Students cried in each other's arms after classes and laboratories, they met in study groups on weekends and evenings. In dissecting lab, Kaas would materialize suddenly to ask, "Why don't you tell me everything you know about the kidney?" If the answer was sufficient, he called the student a "good" boy or girl. One student who had studied ceramics in college dreamed of fashioning a clay mold of the human spleen, then casting a perfect gold replica, which he carried to Dr. Kaas, offering it on bended knees.

On the last day of final exams, there was a Christmas party. A keg of beer ran dry within an hour. Students' faces were sallow but smiling. Without warning, Dr. Kaas appeared and began going from student to student, telling them their exact scores on the final exam. Only one student had not passed, and he stood near the door, stunned.

Four months after that Christmas party, I had dinner with Dr. Kaas. It was spring, a calmer academic quarter, and he was tanned and relaxed after a recent trip to Hawaii. His research on lymphocytes, which he had to neglect each fall to teach anatomy, was going well, he said. As we walked through the evening light toward a restaurant near his laboratory, he talked eagerly about himself. After a childhood in Hungary, he had studied the humanities in gymnasium and had at first been unhappy in medical school, which he completed in England. Before he was too far along in a British surgical practice, he had found time to develop other interests—a deep knowledge of Egyptian history, a wide grasp of literature, and a love for Wagnerian opera. He had left surgery to return to teaching, and he now found medicine to be the "most humanizing factor" in his life.

"The ideal thing," he told me as we reached the restaurant, "is to become hardened enough so that you can deal with situations like cutting into a cadaver—I was very upset when I first saw one—and not lose your sensitivity at other times. Everything in my life follows from this."

Of course, I can't undo myself. I have trained myself to see things. Since I'm interested in art, I can stand in one of the rooms of the National Gallery and I can name you the pictures around the wall. But you can do it too if you give it a little bit of effort—yes, it's perfectly possible. The other thing I specialize in is faces—I like human faces. I can meet somebody downtown and I can remember that I saw that woman buying potatoes next to me in the Safeway two years ago, because she has an interesting face. I am pretty organized in most things I do because I have learned that's the only way I can accomplish half of the things I would like to. And I do consciously try to impress on you that organizing is very important. You can have loose ends hanging around, but the basics of what you learn have to be laid out pretty cold and cut and dried, so that you can lay your hands on them whenever you need to. You've got to achieve a sense of order with what you put into your head, and it's too bad that that intimidates people.

When you get to med school, the learning material is probably different from what you were used to, and you've got to make changes in your attack. There are so many new things, and they pile up, and they all crystallize in the anatomy course, and if I were self-conscious or wanted to go down as the most popular teacher, I wouldn't ask you to achieve as much in your first quarter of school. But it really is good to come down with a bang during that first quarter.

I tell you, Peter, because I care about students during the first quarter. However hard I try, it is impossible not to have some kind of paternalistic feeling toward them. I see a bunch of very good people who are bursting with potential, and I know that they are going to be very good, going to do just fine. And I see them grappling with organization of problems and being snowed under, and my main job is to try and establish some system or routine which will make them cope with this large amount of material being forced on them for the first time.

The easiest way would be to do nothing, to let you go at it and find by your own mistakes what doesn't work and then come up with a system to correct it. But then you will need exactly twice as much time. Do you agree?

You see, there's a basic problem. How do I have the chance in a class of 120 to come across to you, to assure you that it's all right, Peter, to come along with your own system but come, get on with it, do it soon before you get snowed under, and if you don't have the time to work out your own system, for goodness' sake please try mine before you go too far! Now this is being paternalistic. But I have to do this on a large scale, and so I opt for a less than happy medium. I know that 10 or 20 percent of the class will be very antagonistic to the way I have thought out as the best approach. But there is so much to accomplish in that short quarter. By the end of the course, I want to get some kind of confidence into you that you can handle a lot of material, that you can talk about it and organize it. I don't care about the detail—you are going to forget it. I want you to feel at home in the body by the end of the course.

You see, the funny thing about it is that I think anatomy is the most human of all the basic sciences. It is the only part of medicine which deals with the healthy human body. You talk about anything else in medicine, it's always defined in abnormal terms. Take heart sounds. You never hear anybody talk about normal heart sounds except at the very introduction. The basic secret of medicine is that the most difficult thing is to diagnose health. It's very easy to diagnose disease—very, very easy. It's so hard to improve your skill at diagnosing health, and to be able to say what is really normal, and to stand up and defend your judgment by scientific statement that this is what health is. You shouldn't end up practicing medicine with a set bag of tricks. You should evaluate a person's body by a thorough understanding of the workings of it. And that's the anatomy you need. The graduate students who are going to teach anatomy or surgical residents who come back for anatomy courses need to piddle around with all the little details and they don't have to know how the whole structure fits together, but you do, and although at the time you may not feel it fitting together, it sort of becomes part of you and you never have to worry about it—if you have walked through it and it made sense once in your life, that's enough. It would be very easy for me to teach anatomy by turning the lights out and putting up a slide and saying, "Well, this is the greater omentum, and this is the epiploic foramen, and this is such and such a recess"—but why reduce anatomy to rote memorization? Isn't it better instead to take an intellectual approach and try to have you gain a three-dimensional appreciation in your mind?

Of course the problem is how do you cope with an enormous volume of material and crystallize out something which will stay with you for the rest of your life? There is no other way but by hard work, which is painful. The most painful experiences eventually come back with good dividends, you see, and then you are a slightly different animal than you were in the beginning. You become educated, and the definition of education—though most people argue against this—is to change the pattern of behavior. You basically behave differently at the end of the education process than you did at the beginning; you handle material differently, whether it's anatomy or anything else. The gain is only worth its price if the way you behave at the end is better and more efficient. Now with 90 percent of my students, that's probably true. Therefore, I accept the penalty of antagonizing 10 percent of the class who get upset because their personality is too strong. And that's a positive thing, you see, because they're going to survive in any case, whereas the other 80 or 90 percent can use being pushed around and led around and being told what to do—do you see what I mean?

The ideal way for all of this to happen would be if the class was smaller and we had a chance to get to know one another, for me to feel out the individual perspectives. I sense a tremendous barrier to this during the first quarter. It is impossible to get people to come and talk to me before it's almost too late, because you're too damn proud—and you should be at that stage, I mean, you have been doing just terrific, and here comes a stupid anatomy course and it's trying to get you under. So why should you go and talk to somebody? Yet that is the thing you should do, and I can say that until I am blue in the face, it will not happen.

Still, it's very rare that one finds a misfit in medical school—I would say maybe one person per year, not more than that. Occasionally I meet a person who is not cut out for medicine, usually for personal reasons, but it becomes reflected in their academic performance. Because of that poor performance. I begin to look at all the reasons and I see that the picture doesn't fit. Then as I sit in on student-progress committees I see the same person cropping up again and again and I kick myself, saying that I knew that during the first quarter and I should have said so. At the same time, if you get adjusted to my course as you go through it and you feel happy and content at the end of it, I don't think you're going to come across any other part of your medical education which will give you a problem.

Second Year

NANCY SUTERMEISTER, SOPHOMORE MEDICAL STUDENT

Nancy Sutermeister had some time between classes to talk with me. She said with a laugh that one lesson she'd learned in her second year of medical school was that one couldn't study absolutely all the time. We found an unused teaching laboratory on the fifth floor of the medical-school building and sat down among the soapstone-topped microscope cabinets, arching faucets, and chrome gas nozzles.

Nancy seemed instantly as comfortable in the laboratory as she might have been in her home. Thick glasses gave her a studious, mature look, which jarred slightly with her girlish braids and smiling, round face. As she told me of the small town forty miles away where she had grown up, it was clear that she still hadn't adjusted to the city where her medical school was located.

No, she said, she was not a strong feminist. "I have enough on my hands being a medical student and a wife at the same time." Yet she was aware of the growing impact of women on medicine. In 1964, only 8 percent of American medical students were women; by 1977 almost 24 percent were female. Among practicing American physicians in 1977, only one in ten was a woman.

Pausing often at first to phrase her opinions correctly, she soon talked quickly and emotionally about her two loves: medicine and marriage.

"You know, I got rejected the first year that I applied to medical school, and for a while I tried to find something different to do. But medicine is just the perfect career for me—I love patient contact, and I love science. I wouldn't trade this career for anything—I don't care if they don't pay me, I would do it as long as I had a place to live and food, and stuff like that. I really would."

There were a lot of things I didn't like about last year. Many of the classes, like biochemistry, didn't seem pertinent to what I needed to know, but it was okay because I was so happy just to be in medical school, and 'cause I knew that they wanted us to learn the basics. So I kind of went along with it. But this year the classes are all clinical, and I'm totally engrossed in what the lecturers are talking about. We have genetics, and reproductive biology, and musculoskeletal anatomy, and modules where we have four or five lectures on a sub-ject—like anesthesiology or ob-gyn or neurology. Another dif-ference this year is that no one looks over your shoulder to see if you do your homework and get facts straightened out—they trust us a little more. Let's say there's a lecture in neurology and they're talk-ing about ataxias. I remember my neurology from spring quarter of last year, but I don't quite recall how everything fits together in the brain, so if I have some extra time I sit down and work through it again. What's happened to me is that at the end of last year, I sud-denly realized that I was gonna pass my courses. Everybody passes their courses unless they really try to flunk out. Sure, you can get sick or you can have a really difficult time with your personal life so that you flunk a class—but as long as you kind of enjoy them and don't worry too much about the parts you don't like, you get through.

There's also a lot more patient contact this year. We're supposed to spend an afternoon every two weeks either in a physician's office seeing patients or interviewing and doing physicals on patients in a hospital. My first patient had about twenty problems—kidney fail-ure, anemia and bone disease and alcoholism. The patients we're seeing this year are much sicker than the ones I saw last year, I mean really sick. It's hard for me to go into a patient's room when they're that sick. They've already had maybe two histories and phys-icals—from the resident and then from the third- or fourth-year medical student, and now here comes the second-year medical student to do it. I feel intrusive.

Now, you know what happens to me this year? I always get a tension headache. I don't feel nervous or hesitant when I'm working with patients, but I always get a tension headache right in the back of my neck, and every night when I go home I just have to lie down for an hour. There are a lot of expectations that I have to meet. There's the expectations of the patient, and then I've got to go in and present the patient to my tutor, and remember all the things in the physical, making sure that I've gotten all the facts about the disease that's involved, and I've got to do a review of systems and a family history to see if there is any connection. And the patient keeps rambling on. You know, they like to talk a lot so they don't give the information I need; they talk about all these interesting things, but I have to kind of break in—see, I have to be thinking always about my job, what it is that I'm supposed to be doing. It's a tense situation. Then when I'm finished with the patient, I've gotta read Harrison's [textbook of internal medicine], I've gotta look up all the diseases the patient had and thoroughly understand everything.

When I first started working with patients, talking with them and understanding their emotions was real high on my priority list. Now it keeps getting shoved to the bottom. I can see that my tutor does it too, and all the other physicians that I come in contact with—they ask the stock questions that they're supposed to ask: "Well, how do you get along with your husband?" but they don't really listen to what the patient's saying. All that stuff they tell you during the first year about asking open-ended questions and empathizing with patients goes by the wayside, and this year what's important is the medical problem. Yesterday in class, Dr. Barker was presenting a patient with chest pain, and we were going through all of the things that can cause chest pain—how to differentiate—lab tests, physical findings. It's really fun to sit back and think, Well, what are all the things that can cause chest pain? This is what's called the differential diagnosis. Then a guy in our class raised his hand and said, "Well, I really think that we should be worried about this guy's life-style.

You know he's been in jail and he was talking about going out and getting laid."

Everybody laughed, of course, and Dr. Barker said, "What do you mean?" The guy said, "I think we should talk to him about this and maybe do some genito-urinary-tract tests to see if he's got VD and some other things and see if he needs any help with his personal life." And Dr. Barker says, "Well, I know there's something called family medicine, but I think that's a little bit far out."

After all, the medical problem is what you're there to learn, and if you're wrapped up in what the patients are feeling and what's going on in their personal life it takes away from concentrating on the medical problem. It's not that it's not important, but as a student you can't—you're not going to be able to help a patient unless you learn the medicine too.

You might like to hear about a patient I had last year. I went in to take his medical history, and he'd had a prostatectomy—his prostate removed—and I knew I should ask him if he'd had any side effects— problems with going to the bathroom or sexual function. And he told me, "Oh, yeah," and he started talking about his problems. He said he couldn't have intercourse with his wife after this surgery, but he said that he could get an erection. It kind of rang a bell for me, because if he could get an erection there was no excuse for him not to have intercourse with his wife. And you wouldn't believe the problems this guy had. I spent an hour and a half on his personal history. He was a child molester and had been in a psychiatric hos- pital for eighteen months. He wasn't a homosexual, but he had always been attracted to male children and had had sexual relations with a couple of them—twelve and thirteen years old—and then he was found out, and he really hated himself for doing this and went to a psychiatric hospital but didn't get any help at all. He started crying when he was telling me this story. I, I felt very sorry for this person, and I really felt he needed a lot of help and that his emotional problems were much more severe than his medical problems, and they weren't being looked at at all. I went out and read the chart on him and there was absolutely nothing about what was really his problem, and I was really mad. So I skipped class to talk to my tutor because I was so upset. Do you know what he said to me? He kind of stepped back and listened to the whole story, and after I finished he said, "Nancy, you know you wouldn't have spent an hour and a half talking to someone about their cold." He said, "Do you see how being a physician can be very voyeuristic?" I just—I was so mad. He said he felt that lots of times I asked questions which were really not pertinent to the history, that I was being nosy and in a way voyeuristic. It made me have a bad feeling about medicine.

I was thinking yesterday when I was leaving school that the women medical students complain about everything. They complain about the classes, they complain about professors, they complain about not sleeping and getting fat and studying too much. But I've noticed that the men are much quieter—they just kind of do the work and accept it as being the way it is, as if there was only one way to do it. With the women, I can always bring up some subject and then bellyache about it, and we'll laugh and joke about it and most of the men will look at me like I'm nuts. So maybe I just enjoy bellyaching.

What's my schedule like? Well, I usually study one or two hours before eight-thirty, before my pharmacology class, and then two or three hours before my afternoon classes, and then either none or one or two hours in the evening. I'd rather take time off piecemeal, so I try and keep my evenings free. Tom, my husband, and I can go to a show, or watch TV, or go visit my brother, who lives in the city. I'd rather have evenings free than study all week and take weekends off. Still, I usually take Saturday afternoons off completely, after my morning class. Sundays are sacred. I don't want any visitors, I kind of get rid of my husband—you know, he goes and sees a game on TV or something—and I get up and I study for three or four hours in the morning, and read the paper, and have a quiet breakfast, maybe light a fire in the fireplace and read a little bit and kind of relax in the afternoon, studying off and on while I do the laundry and some other things that have to get done. Sunday's the best day.

I don't keep up with too many friends from outside of school. It's not that I study all the time, but when I have free time off I either want to be by myself or I want to do something with Tom. I used to feel guilty—like on Saturday night when someone had asked us to go to a party, and I knew I wasn't gonna study that night, but I still didn't want to go, because when you go to school six days a week and you've gotta study on Sunday, you just don't like to spend free time with other people—you need some peaceful time. Tom understands the situation, and he'll call up the friends and say over the phone, "Nancy just can't come, God, she'd really like to, but she has to study." Last year I always came to school in the morning to study, and when it got close to exams I'd stay at school in the evening and study with different people. And I would get really depressed because I'd think, "Gee, I haven't been home, and I haven't seen Tom," and soon I'd be depressed to the point where I couldn't even study the next day.

See, now I'm at the point where I'm doing the work because I know I need to do it. I'm not doing it to pass the course. I feel a certain responsibility to learn the material, and so I do what it takes to get done, which means really limiting my life. But time with Tom is crucial to me, partly because he has multiple sclerosis—did I tell you that? Yeah—MS. It's a degenerative disease, but there are all different degrees of it. We've been married for five years, and two or three years before we got married he had symptoms on and off, and then the year after we got married he was student teaching and working too hard, and he really got sick. So he quit working, and got much better. The main reason is that he doesn't exert himself. He's got a really good doctor down in Portland. Before that he was referred to all these different ophthalmologists and neurologists for this bizarre symptoms, and all the physicians thought he had MS, but no one of them would diagnose it, because there's really not a whole lot they can do for it.

But this doctor in Portland—it's real weird—he treats the disease with a diet—a low-fat diet. You know, immediately you think, ha, ha, a real quack. But this guy isn't a quack. He was head of neurology at Oregon State Medical School for twenty years, and he found during the war that when everyone else was really, really sick because they couldn't get meat and dairy products, MS patients got better. You know, I was basically a scientist before I got into medical school. I was involved in research biochemistry, and my science teachers instilled certain attitudes in me, so I would never say that just because Tom's doing better that doctor is right. But I also know that there's a lot of placebo effect involved in patients who have MS, because your nervous system is sick, and if the nervous system is optimistic, it does better all around. But then when they talk about MS in neurology class, they present it as a really bleak, incurable disease. And then the first patient I saw in my neurology preceptorship had MS. That was hard to take, because I had helped Tom come to the conclusion that he's not really an MS patient. Well, he does have MS, but he's okay, you know. Then for me to see this neurology patient who probably was fine ten years ago, but who is now very sick and probably isn't gonna get a whole lot better—it was hard to take. It was difficult to stick Tom into the category of "yeah, he really does have MS, and all these things could happen." That was pretty hard to take, you know.

The week after we talked, I ran into Nancy in the small student lounge adjacent to the room lined with study carrels. She was helping to set up the second-year class's presentation of skits about medical school.

"Hey, there," she called out, "would you like to help us? We need someone to impersonate our reproductive-biology instructor. Do you know any good flashers?" She and the other students in charge were giggling, handing out props to the hastily comandeered cast, and writing impromptu jokes on paper usually used for taking medical histories. Later that day the same jokes rolled out, one after another, as the room full of students, faculty, and administrators roared with laughter. There were jokes about incompetent lecturers, about the names given to cadavers, about burn victims being called "crispy critters," about terminal cases in the cancer ward being called GORKS: God Only Really Knows. There were few jokes about women, and none about multiple sclerosis.

Third Year

BRIAN O'MALLEY, JUNIOR MEDICAL STUDENT

At the end of the second year, medical students take the National board exams—two days of standardized testing reminiscent of the MCATs. Many schools make a passing grade on the National Boards a prerequisite for credit for the first two years of instruction. Yet most students pass on either the first or second try, and soon afterward they begin their third-year clerkships. Most of the third year is taken up by the "big five" required clerkships: obstetrics and gynecology, pediatrics, psychiatry, internal medicine, and surgery. Each takes between six and twelve weeks to complete.

One black, unruly lock of Brian O'Malley's hair was constantly falling over his high forehead. This accented the way he had of taking a half-step back and casting a critical look at the world around him. When we talked, that world was for him dominated by his surgery clerkship at a Veterans Administration hospital in a western city.

Of all the required clerkships, surgery has the most formidable reputation. Some students relish the intensity, others hate it. Two months before I talked with Brian, one of his classmates had jumped off a high bridge during a surgery clerkship at another hospital.

It was Saturday noon, and Brian had just attended his weekly didactic session at the medical school. Now it was time for him to get back to the VA hospital and check on his patients. We walked across freshly cut lawns to the entrance of the imposing brick building, set by itself on a hill above the city.

The stark lobby was almost empty, and when we reached the

sixth floor, the surgery ward, the only activity was an old man groggily negotiating the corridor in pajamas. The day nurse looked up from some paperwork at the ward desk as Brian walked up to her.

"Hello, Doctor O'Malley," she said. Brian didn't bother to correct her. He asked for any news on the patients. There was little, since many had checked out on weekend passes. The operating room at the end of the ward was darkened behind windowed double doors. The principal sounds came from radios and televisions playing through their own static in the patients' rooms opening onto the hall.

Brian went into the staff office and took a white coat off the rack. When he put it easily on, I could see that the name tag was almost identical to a doctor's.

There was some "scut work" to do, Brian told me after reading a note from his resident on the bulletin board. There were some orders for medications to check on and record in the patients' medical charts, and some blood samples to draw. He walked back to the nursing station and entered the storeroom, lined with shelves and racks for dressings, tools, bedpans, and miscellaneous equipment. Rummaging through a cardboard box of glass vials, Brian called out to the nurse, "Are we using red-top blood tubes this week?"

In a room down the hall, a veteran was sitting in bed picking at his lunch, his folds of skin blending with the bedclothes. Brian stopped at the door, needles and vials in hand.

"I'm sorry, Mr. Duarte. I didn't know you were eating. I'll come back when you're through. I'd hate to spoil your appetite with a blood test." Three old men in the other beds around the room nodded approvingly, then went back to watching soap operas on their overhead television sets.

"Let's get some lunch ourselves," Brian said, walking back toward the elevator. "The cafeteria will be a good place to talk."

In the privacy of a cafeteria booth, with soothing music drifting down from the ceiling speakers, Brian began to draw together thoughts and impressions from the past three weeks.

If we have forty patients and our first surgery is scheduled for eight
o'clock, we'll have rounds at six A.M. Before rounds I have to go and
see every patient and amass all of the data from the night before.
That usually means looking at the chart—do they have a fever?—
looking at the oral input, looking at the urinary output, any drainage
coming out of any tubes, make sure everything is unplugged, making sure that nobody has crashed during the night. If any blood
needs to be drawn, I'll do it, if any IVs need to be started, I'll do it.
Obviously, nobody sits and talks to the patient; if the patient is
asleep you don't even wake him up, you just run around. Sometimes I'll be in there drawing blood and the patient will start off on a
war story, and I know if I stayed around to listen I'd hear some great
war stories, but there's too much else to do. Besides, it's dangerous
to get too empathetic—I learned this back when I was working my
first emergency room. A patient came in and she was bleeding
because she had cut her hand, and already I'd seen a couple of guys
come in with cut hands and it hadn't bothered me, but this woman
was obviously in pain. She was really hurting, and I could em-
pathize with her so much. I was just watching what the doctor was
doing, and then all of a sudden she would cry out with pain. He
hadn't anesthetized her quite enough and she was having trouble
tolerating the stitches. Suddenly my skin went white and I broke
out in a cold sweat, and I could feel the blood rushing out of my
head, and I had to get up and leave the room, so I didn't learn much
from that. I talked it over later with the doc, who is a friend of mine,
and he said, "Look, the only way you can beat this game is don't em-
pathize with the patient—you just can't do that." The danger of it is
that you can stop feeling for the patients at all. You never put yourself in their place; you come to identify with the profession and get
all your strokes from other docs, and that's what's happening in this
place: the students depend on the residents, the residents depend
on the students, everybody depends on the senior doctor, and the
patients are just grist for the mill.

A lot of mornings before rounds I just look at what the nurses
have written and take for granted that what they've written is true.

Frequently, though, I find that the nurses fabricate things like the patient's weight. They look in and say, "Oh, well, he probably hasn't changed from yesterday, and I don't want to bring the scale all the way in here, I've got too many other things to do." A lot of critical numbers get lost at the VA, because the nurses don't write them down. The perennial problem is with somebody who has got a catheter on, and it slips off, and none of that is written down, and then someone attending comes by and says, "This patient's urinary output has been down every day for three days," and in fact that's not the case.

You can't trust anything—you have to do everything yourself. We order bloods and they never get drawn—the paperwork is all done and you never realize until the slip doesn't come back that no blood was drawn. It's so aggravating to see nurses bucking responsibility. What they'll do is grab the student and say, "Look, this hasn't been done," when the reason it hasn't been done is that either the nurse or the ward secretary didn't do their job, and their way of covering up for it is to get the medical student to track it down for them. Students make this system work, but the question is "Do I want to make it work?"

Of course some of the very good nurses get burned out in this place, because they have too many patients to care for, and they don't have adequate training for the tasks they are asked to do. Plus, this is a real cantankerous population of patients. They tend to order people around; they're not the nicest patients to work with. They're Skid Row types—people who've been in the military and who never made it in the world. Some of them just come here to pick up some prescriptions, or if they have some major surgery, but the vast majority are the seriously ill vets who have been down and out on their luck for twenty years—chronic smokers and advanced alcoholics, and a whole lot of them are crazy. Since they closed the mental hospitals in the state and put everybody onto the street, they check into VA hospitals as hotels.

It was worse for me when I first came on the service and had to care for forty patients I had never seen before. I had no idea what their electrolytes were like the day before, since there hadn't been any med students to record it for five days, in between the shifts, and the patients had been floundering, and one resident had the responsibility for forty patients, at least six of whom were in intensive care. Where I'm at right now is very different. I've honed my skills and learned the system, and I'm doing pretty well. I mean yesterday the ward secretary complimented me because I had all of her work done, I had all of the nurses' work done, and all of my work done, and it was only four o'clock in the afternoon!

We use the team system here. A team will consist of one or two med students, an intern, and a resident. The philosophy on our team is that we work together to get the work done so that we can go home. The idea is that whoever's free does it. There's usually two of us in the operating room at any time. Sometimes there are three of us, so that philosophy gets us by. In the OR, students are usually holding retractors and peering over the surgeon's shoulder. Occasionally you might get to sew up, but I did a lot more sewing on my obstetrics clerkship—episiotomies and C sections. Here I've closed midline incisions and stitched up a few laparotomies, which are pretty easy.

The most crucial working relationship is between the intern and the student, and so much of that is personality. On my very first clerkship I started off with a bad intern, but then he left and I got a good one so that I could see the contrast, and I said, "Shit, I don't have to put up with that." Interns are the ones who appreciate you most, because if you can help them with their work and help them get home sooner, they love you. And a lot of the jobs which to them are scut work are still interesting to me. I need practice drawing blood, and practice putting in IVs, and practice working up patients, and practice going through all of the charts to find things. Reading through a seven- or eight-pound chart—I don't know how you quantify charts, but they are big—you can see the flow of the disease, and you can discover things others have overlooked. I spent about two hours the other day going through a chart and found out that it had been assumed that the patient's seizures had been lifelong. I discovered that in fact they were caused by trauma in 1971, and the doc who was taking care of him two months ago dropped one of his antiseizure medications. The rationale for dropping the medication may have been that the guy was in renal failure, but it was never entered in the chart. The medication was there one week and gone the next, and the guy seized while in physical therapy, so we put him back on the medication. That's the quality of care.

When I'm on call—around here that means every third night—I usually get a few hours' sleep after work is finished, but the nurses call you at their whim and convenience to do things any hour of the night. I may get up and draw blood, or start an IV, or change somebody's dressings: that's very critical. It has to be done with aseptic technique. One lady had a graft that had been done three times before and had never taken, so we did it again, and it really made the difference in whether she would be able to keep that leg or not. The graft got infected postsurgery, and it was absolutely mandatory that perfect sterile technique be done on the dressing changes, so it was delegated to the medical students to do that! Even though I did not know the patient and I had never done a dressing change before, because I was the student, I did it. I was supposed to have gone in with the previous student and seen how to do it, but because of the time crunch, the other student described it to me in thirty seconds, and I went and did it.

That's one of the great frustrations at the VA: nobody shows you how to do something, you learn by doing. It's scary when you come onto the wards and the rest of the staff assumes that you're the best one in the hospital at drawing blood, just because you keep sticking the patient until you get a vein. On a couple of occasions I have told people that I just couldn't get it, but there are some students that won't do that—they'll just keep sticking them. You have to be fairly aggressive, that's the party line, but the thing I dislike most about the VA, and the reason I resisted being assigned here, is that the patients are treated as practice material in this hospital. There are a lot of them, they're elderly, they're alcoholic, they're poor, they're in for multiple problems, and while there are attending staff here for some of the major surgery, most of the responsibility and management goes to second-year residents. The responsibility gets shoved down, and things have been happening which have really upset me.

A lot of the surgery here is plastic surgery—removing growths, doing skin grafts. The plastic surgeon is supposed to be here supervising, and the interns are supposed to be there, but they don't come. Last week there were maybe fifteen or twenty patients who came in to have something excised, and students who had never done excisions before in their lives went in and excised these things. We had a case—a pedicle graft—where the patient had a huge growth on his forehead—possibly cancerous, probably not, but the growth had to be excised. The attending surgeon came in and drew a line with blue ink on the guy's head, described how to cut it, and then left. A medical student who had never done anything like this before did it. There was another medical student in the room who had been a corpsman in Vietnam who had a little bit more knowledge about surgical technique. He had been in a lot of rooms where it was going on, and after the other student was already closing, he mentioned to her that maybe she should irrigate underneath the wound, to get the blood out. I guess this is standard procedure, but I had never heard of it before myself.

The same patient came back in this week, and it looks like the graft may not take. Now this could mean that the guy is going to have a hole in his head the size of a baseball. Of course he's an elderly guy, and his face. . . . It's not going to make a hell of a lot of cosmetic difference, and if it has to be grafted it will be grafted, but when all this was going on, the surgeon who should have been supervising was down the hall!

This week I asked the resident to come down, and he did, because we were going to take some xanthomas—little cholesterol deposits—off of someone's face and eyes, and I wanted to learn how to do that because it's kind of a nifty thing to do, and it's relatively safe and simple. So I volunteered to work with him on this, and right in the middle of the procedure he got called out to go to the operating room, and all he had done was put in the anesthetic. The plastic surgeon came in and said, "Do you want to do this?" And I said yes, so he said, "Okay, here's how you do it," and he drew three lines on a piece of paper and said, "This is how you make your incision. Follow the skin lines; this is how you sew it up. Now, good luck." And then he left, and I took out the xanthomas, and the resident never came back until I was almost finished, and then all he said was "That looks pretty good." Well, I am scared shitless that I may have broken my aseptic technique and that the patient may come back with an infected face! She's a fiftyish lady, she has really elastic skin, it was an easy closure and will probably heal, but my father had the same operation done by a plastic surgeon, and this poor woman got a third-year medical student who had never done it before. This is the way the VA system works. A lot of students like to come to the VA precisely because they get to do so much, but my argument is that people should not be discriminated against merely because they are poor and they're taking advantage of free medical care.

The students had a big discussion about this situation last week, and I was the odd man out. I told the other students that we shouldn't have been doing what we did, that it's wrong. One student said to me, "Brian, if you persist in this kind of attitude, you're going to be a bad doctor, because you're not aggressive enough." He said, "This is the best time to do these procedures, while we're students and the hospital and med school are covering our asses if something goes wrong." In a way, that student was right—if I don't do procedures I'll never learn them, but it's really Hitleresque. We can do these things because someone orders us to do it, and the chain of responsibility provides insurance.

They've got us scared of admitting incompetence, of asking for help with a procedure. You can say, "I don't know," but if you do that too much, the system comes down on you. One of our professors told us last week, "There's a big gray area out there where the decisions aren't easy, and someday you'll have to deal with it on your own."

Fourth Year

STEVE SEIGEL, SENIOR MEDICAL STUDENT

By the fourth year of medical school, most of the required clerkships have been completed, and there is time for electives, for looking into various facets of the profession in more depth. As a subintern, a fourth-year student can receive almost as much responsibility for a number of patients as a true intern does.

Fourth year is also when decisions about the next few years become imminent. Most students choose to apply for internship and residency training in one of the twenty-two recognized specialties, and begin visiting programs at the end of the third year. They soon come into contact with the nationwide computer service which matches students' preferred residencies with each hospital training program's list of acceptable applicants.

Steve Seigel was only two months away from receiving his M.D. when we talked in a dim corner of a bar not far from his medical school. He arrived and unshouldered his books, and when the waitress came by, he ordered a pitcher of beer, his eyes gleaming as he said the word. He wore a basketball jersey, threadbare from much use, and when he spoke, an athletic vitality and optimism pervaded his words. His wiry blond curls were thinning, and this made him look older than his twenty-six years. When I asked him a question, his steady grin would give way to a squint. Then he would scratch his head, lean forward grasping his beer glass, and share his perceptions with me.

I'm kind of in limbo right now, waiting for the results of the match, which should come out in two weeks. That's the day where every-

thing is on the line but it's out of your hands. By signing up and join-
ing the match program, you're committed to accept whatever residency is offered to you. You know, you've got your list of
preferences in, and then the computer tells you where you're gonna
be for the next five years. I'm looking at surgery, with an interest in
urology. This will probably mean doing two years of general surgery
and then reapplying for another residency in urology, four more
years. I'm looking at programs in LA, Phoenix, and San Diego,
since I want to be on the West Coast.

In this education game it seems you're always working your way
to the top just to get knocked down again. You know, you're the big
high-school senior and then boom, you're only a college freshman;
then you graduate from college, you think you're a big king and go
to med school, and you're right back at the bottom. Right now I'm a
fourth-year med student, and I feel like I actually know something,
but next year I'll have to do all the work no one else wants to do.

Medicine is very unusual. I don't think most professions have
anything like a match system, where you're pretty much guaranteed
a job. The only problem is that you're forced to make a decision
early about what field you want to go into, and you never know how
you come to do it. I look at my friends who are going into pediatrics,
and ob-gyn, and psychiatry, and pathology, and some I would have
predicted, and some I would never have guessed. A lot of my
friends were saying that I'd never go into surgery. When I tell them
it's definite they kind of step back and say, "God, but you're so easy-
going, how can you go into surgery?" Then they say, "Well, I hope
surgery doesn't change you."

I think everyone comes into med school very different, with lots
of sharp corners to their personality, and through med school those
corners get squared off to some degree, even though everyone tries
to hold on to some individuality. We all hold on to something, but
just to function in medicine you've gotta throw away some of your
idealism. Take welfare, for instance. I used to have a lot of liberal
ideas about it. But I did my medicine clerkship at the county hospital, and I saw people on welfare call up the ambulance just to bring
them in for a cold. There are lots of little things like that which have

made me much more cynical. I majored in psychology in college
and really wanted to do something in medicine that involved counseling and psychology. Originally, I planned to go into pediatrics.
But during my clerkships I saw that so much of medicine is treating
social disease. At the county hospital, people come in night after
night just for alcoholic detoxification, or because they fell over
again, or get punched out. I would see their charts getting bigger
and bigger with every admission, but the individual patient would
hardly ever change. We'd fix them up and put them back on the
street, and they'd roll right back in the following week. And working
in these situations I'd have to do things that no one would do out of
choice. I mean, no one would get up and see these people at three
in the morning, and touch them—you know? It's such grunge work.
It's just amazing what I found I could put up with, but I decided that
primary care was not for me as a profession. You think you're doing
medicine, but what you're really dealing with is the problems of society. That county hospital would close down, in my opinion, if it
weren't for alcoholism and related diseases, and alcoholism is a
social problem, not a medical problem.

So, yeah, I got disillusioned. I did pathology at the same county
hospital, and I got to see another side of medicine. I'd be sitting at a
medical-morbidity conference, where we'd debate the cause of a patient's death, only I'd have the autopsy report, and I'd know the
cause of death, and then I'd see the internists come in and spend
hours doing what I call shadowboxing. In other words, they'd go
through the differential diagnosis and pick the most bizarre disease
and try to see how they could get the patient to have died of that
cause. Internal medicine is like that. You go through the entire differential and you try to rule this out and rule that out, and instead of
ruling in anything you spend all your time ruling out.

Sure, in surgery you go through a differential, but you always go
after what is on top of your list first, and as long as the patient
doesn't get worse, you continue along that line. What's more, with
surgery, you make a diagnosis, and then you *do* something. You
take on a case, and in an organized way you make somebody sick in
order to make them well, while all the internal-medicine people

ask, "Why don't you get this test first?" or "Why don't you wait another week?" and you really think that if you operate now you can save the patient money in the long run, and provide for their health right now. Surgeons' personalities probably seem aggressive and abrasive to someone who is more laid-back, because surgeons want to be on the move. Things happen a lot faster in surgery; there's not always time to think about all the possibilities.

Also, I think—I don't know what this is going to sound like, but I think other doctors are jealous of surgeons, because of all the procedures that they get to do. When you're doing a medicine clerkship, you don't talk about how many pages of Harrison's you've read, or how many cases of Lupus erythematosus you *saw*, but you'll say, "Well, I got to do a lumbar puncture today," or "I've done three bone marrows." Well, a surgeon does that all the time. He'll do the procedures, and I think he'll keep that youthful, med-student attitude about wanting to do the procedures himself. He doesn't want anyone else curing his patients. I think people knock surgeons because they feel like the surgeon jumps in, takes the procedure out of their hands, does something definitive and fun, and then leaves. A lot of people resent that.

Besides, the surgeons I've met are much more down-to-earth than most doctors. They get involved, and they work in teams. The surgeon might have the ultimate say, but without the scrub nurses and the anesthesiologists and the OR technicians and the med students, they couldn't get anything done. It's like pickup basketball, which I love. I'll go down to the intramurals building and get into a pickup game, and just play, and lose myself in the game. I'm always amazed at how eight guys who don't know each other can walk onto a court with a little hoop and play organized games, and try to help each other out to win a ball game, and then it's over, and we leave.

I did two subinternships in surgery to find out what it would be like. As a subintern I really had the responsibility of an intern. I had my own patients and wrote orders for them. I was able to function as an intern without quite the same power, and I got to see what the hours are like. When you're on call you've gotta be able to react to a problem almost instantaneously, and you learn to be real efficient.

When you're on call you've always gotta let people know where you are. You gotta take your bellboy in with you even when you take a shit, in case the nurses call you. On my subinternship, I'd go to sleep with the phone hanging about six inches from my ear on the wall, and when that phone went off, I would pick it up and the nurse would start talking, and I'd say, "Just wait a second," and then "Okay, go ahead and repeat that." You've got to wake up, but it's actually amazing what you can do. One thing about surgery is that I really surprised myself. I used to think that if I didn't get seven to eight hours of sleep I would be no good, but now I find that I can be good for thirty-six hours without any sleep. Maybe toward the end I'm not as sharp, but I can function, I can do my job, though I won't be at my most energetic. I won't be joking with nurses. It gets down to strictly business—I want to get the work done and get out.

I've learned to not waste time when I work. I can do the physical, the history, and the review of systems all at once when I'm working up a patient. I've got it down to where I can go bang, bang, bang, you know, writing while I'm talking and doing the physical. I'll examine the head and ask "Have you had any headaches?" then I'll look in the ears: "Or ringing in your ears?" I just keep moving along like that, writing things down as I go.

What's weird about being on call is coming home after it's over. A lot of times I'll walk out and have forgotten where I parked my car, because I parked it two days before. I'll go home and there will be two-day-old papers, and letters, and stuff waiting for me to do. All of a sudden a few days have gone by, then a few weeks, and I never got to the bank, my bills are late—it's incredible. Actually, it's almost weirder being on call inside the hospital and having nurses and staff come rolling in from the outside, talking and seeming fresh, and I'll realize all of a sudden that I've been there all night, and the people I saw go home the day before are just coming back to work, and I haven't left. But that's the key difference about being a professional. Nurses have a profession but I don't call them professionals, because when their eight-hour shift is over, they're gone. They don't have to wait until a problem is solved. They'll say, "Sorry, it's three o'clock, I've gotta go." A doctor wouldn't even think of saying that.

In general surgery, I'll be on call either every other night, or every third night. It depends on the service. I'll probably do a month of being on every other night, and then a month of being on every third. It's incredible to think that I'll get paid maybe $12,000 a year, and put in 120 hours a week, which works out to less than two dollars an hour. If you want to make money, you shouldn't go into medicine, though I suppose it gives you some job security. But I'm pretty happy with the money, I mean I'm getting a new car, which I couldn't have afforded as a student.

What's my social life like right now? Well, I intend to get married, but now's not the time. In medicine you take it as you can get it, which is why so many medical students end up going out with nurses. Most of my friends in school are going out with people in the health-care field. My best friend is going out with a nurse from the county hospital, and I'm going out with a nurse from neurosurgery. It's just the kind of people you meet on a day-to-day basis. Before I might have said I wanted to go out with someone in music or the arts so that I could forget about medicine and talk about other things, but how often do you meet someone in art if you work in a hospital thirty-six hours straight? The people you're up all night with are the people who get to know you well. So I kind of put up with this. I don't know if it's ideal, but that's the way it is. The thing that scares me the most is the number of doctors who get divorced—higher than the rest of the population.

I have this girl friend in town, but I couldn't ask her to come with me next year. I just couldn't subject anyone to that, you know? If things looked surprisingly good I could always call and say, "Would you come down here?" but I couldn't think of dragging anyone out of their environment to sit at home while I was at the hospital, or to try and get a new job in a city where they might see me ten or twenty hours out of the week, and I might be asleep for fifteen hours out of that twenty. So I feel pretty happy to be single. I don't need the extra hassle on my time. I want to be able to stay late if I have to stay late without having to call in or disappoint someone.

So, yeah, it will be hard for the next few years, but it will be fun. When I was interviewing for different programs, I'd talk to the interns and see how they were liking it. At the best places, the interns were what I'd describe as "smiley tired"—they were working their butts off, and they were happy with the situation. Nowhere is it gonna be easy. I can just write that off, but I'm looking for a place where it will be manageable, where I can really learn something and have a good time. The two years will go fast, I'm sure. At times like this, when I sit here in this tavern having a beer with you, I think of how rare this is gonna be for the next few years, and the future doesn't seem too appealing. But I know I'll get into it. I enjoy being busy, I really do.

PART II

Training

"See one, do one, teach one."

—Medical Proverb

Almost all medical graduates enter a residency after earning their M.D. degrees. A license to practice medicine requires at least one year of postgraduate training. A residency *is* training, not education. There is no time for the "whys" of medicine—there is too much to learn about "how."

As a resident, one is a member of the "house staff" of a hospital. The hospital has become a house in the sense that a resident may spend more hours there each week than anywhere else. A neurosurgeon thought back twenty years to his own residency. "I started in July and didn't leave the hospital grounds again until November, even though I was married. Another member of the house staff covered for me while I went to a Yale–Dartmouth football game. I was so smashed on booze by half-time that I didn't come to until the following day. Fortunately, my friend was covering for me all night."

But it is a regimented house—the lines of command are clearly drawn. The interns, junior residents, and senior residents—or "R Ones, R Twos, and R Threes"—answer to each other by order of seniority, and to a more senior chief resident, who is responsible to the attending physicians and the director of the residency program. Everyone interacts, but the rigid protocols allow the practice of full-time medicine to overshadow questions of authority. "Everything is very straightforward," a woman surgical resident said over the phone, a strong hint of exhaustion in her voice. "There's no time for anything but medicine, no chance to be distracted by anything outside of the hospital. My priorities are so clear. The intensity of the learning makes it worthwhile."

When Flexner was championing four-year medical schools, most physicians served only a year-long internship before beginning practice. Yet with the growth of hospitals and the geometric increase in medical knowledge, three- and four-year residencies became the rule. A specialized residency, such as one in neurosurgery, can last up to six years. "But never again," an attending physician reminded me, "will you be so close to the forefront of modern medicine." A study showed that residents tended to be far better than practicing doctors at correctly prescribing drugs. And an economic study by the AMA showed that house staff keep down hospital costs by providing cheap skilled labor.

"On call" schedules vary. The house staff is running the hospital, and this means that all-night shifts are frequent. "Every other night"—thirty-six hours on, twelve off, thirty-six on, twelve off is widespread, especially in surgical residencies, where it can last through the five years of a surgeon's training. Every other night on call means that the resident is working roughly 120 hours a week— and a week is only 168 hours long!

Almost every doctor I talked with, young and old, had some vivid stories to tell about his residency years. As is true of war stories I heard certain themes over and over—the working past the point of exhaustion, the intense camaraderie of the house staff, the terrible blunders, and the exhilarating successes. For all the eye rolling and black humor, however, few thought that the system of training was wrong, that it could or should be changed. It was a necessary evil— an obstacle course to look back on with even a bit of nostalgia.

Even when I told them about scientific studies that showed how mandatory, repetitive sleep deprivation caused widespread depression and other psychological disturbances, how it impaired learning and functioning ability, they shook their heads.

"You'll never know what it's like," exulted one resident, "until you've been past the point of exhaustion so many times that medicine becomes a spinal reflex, so that when you've been working forty hours straight and take a nap for half an hour, and the nurse wakes you up because there's a code [a cardiac arrest], you go to work, and as you start to move you feel a rush go through your body and pretty soon you are a pure, switched-on, medical machine."

And as an R Two in surgery said, looking ahead to three more years of being on call every other night: "The only trouble with every other night on is that I miss half the cases!"

Intern Year

Intern, from the Latin *internus*, meaning interior.

They hunched over a table in the noisy hospital cafeteria, cradling their cups of coffee and blinking in the slanting morning light coming through plate-glass windows. Nick Peters, a lanky man in his late twenties with a shock of unruly hair falling over his hairline, which was starting to recede, had just finished his morning rounds on the surgery ward, where he had been working for the last three weeks. It was part of his general exposure to the vast field of pediatric medicine. Nick's buddy Ray Winn had been up all night caring for patients, and had twelve hours left before he could go home. Ray was a dark, compact man with a trace of a southern accent in his measured, reassuring voice. The humor and openness with which he spoke balanced Nick's wry talk of frustration. Both men wore their stethoscopes around their necks like thin scarves of rubber tubing and chrome. Attached to their belts were the ever present "beepers," the electronic paging devices. As long as they were wearing them, the hospital switchboard could page them anywhere within a two- or three-mile radius of the hospital.

As they talked about the progress of the year so far, their voices became intense. There was a lot they wanted to say.

N. We'll both be done with the intern year next month, and that's a relief. Most of the year you are on call every third night, so when you go home after being on call, you've been up all night and you go to sleep early because you're exhausted.

R. The next night you go to sleep early because you're going to be on the next night.

N. That's right—you sort of get ready for the onslaught. But part of the year you are on every fourth night, and then you can stay up late the second night because the next night you won't have to be on.

R. It's great to have someone at home, someone to come home to. You don't get home the nights you're on call, the next night you go home and crash, and the next night you can say "Hi!" and make babies, stuff like that. When you're on call, you work thirty-six, thirty-four hours and your brain shuts off.

N. I don't know, I find that when I get tired I just get angrier and angrier. I begin to say, "Goddam, why am I here?"

R. Yeah, but there's always something that's got to get done. Say you're on all night, and you've got a lot of sick patients, and then you've got to be with them the next day. Chances are the kids' parents will be there, and they can tell how tired you are. But there's a lot of sympathy for us from those parents. You like people to think you're working hard; it makes you feel good when they say, "You look terrible!" You want to squeeze everybody and say thank you, but you try and suppress that—it's a very rude thing to do. The parents aren't expecting you to hug them, right? That's really hard sometimes. In med school they spent all this time trying to teach us how to deal with being flirted with, or having the move put on us, but it has never happened to me.

N. It happened to me with one kid's mother, but the only reason she was doing it was that she was so uptight. This was . . . uh . . . God, my mind. . . . I'm just lost today. Benji's mom, that was it, but she really didn't mean it, she just wasn't crazy about having him in here, and thought that if she got real chummy, got in good with the house staff, she would know what was going on better. Benji was in with chronic lung disease and spent some time in the intensive-care unit.

R. That's a creepy room. There are people who work in intensive care for a year and a half or more, and that's just stupid, that's too much. What is scary for me is walking into a place like that and having to take over a lot of patients right away.

N. Really.

R. But I'm starting to feel that there are only a certain number of things you can do in any situation. At first I looked at a problem and said, "Oh my God, what am I going to do?" Now I'm starting to turn around and say, "These are things I *can* do, and how many of them apply to this situation?" I'm not very good at it yet; it's something you evolve into, almost like rote memory. You know, CBC count is so and so; does this kid need antibiotics or does he need to be tapped; does he need Xrays. All instead of saying, "There's a problem here and this looks wrong here. . . ."

N. Yeah, what's the differential diagnosis and how do I exclude each of those differentials? [laugh]

R. There's no way to do that because in the middle of the night there is a patient brought in and you have to do something in a flash. And if you don't know what to do, it is scary.

N. I've come to feel more comfortable saying, "I don't know what's going on," and calling up whoever I need to for advice. The support system feels a lot more familiar than it did in the beginning of the year, and that makes a big difference—knowing who to call.

R. Yeah, when you start in the fall, your first idea is to call somebody, but they don't know who the hell you are, and they treat you like you don't know anything. But now we can call anybody we want to and they will know us and say, "Oh yeah, I'll help you out."

N. This isn't true at a lot of programs. I know it's not true in Boston, and one of the reasons we didn't go to Denver was the third-year residents who said that other doctors were just beginning to know who they were.

R. I'm from Alabama, and before I came here I looked at a lot of other places, mostly in the Southwest and the West Coast, and this place was the best.

N. Have you ever spent much time on the East Coast?

R. Never ever been there.

N. You know what would be great? You want to take a trip to the East Coast when we are done here?

R. Sure!

N. I grew up in New Jersey and went to college and medical at Harvard. You know, for a while I considered graduate school in urban planning at Harvard.

R. Incredible! I just can't believe the number of things you've done!

N. Look where they've all led now! The place they've led me to is nice, but what a life!

R. Speaking of jobs, you know Jim Anderson, that private doctor in Chehalis?

N. I know his name.

R. Really nice guy. I told him one of these days I was going to come down and visit him. And he said, "I'll sign you up."

N. Did he?

R. No, it was just an off-the-cuff thing.

N. You have to go a couple hours' drive to find a lot of pediatric opportunities, because there is a real glut in the city.

R. Who wants to practice in the city?

N. I would!

R. Who wants to be a slug in the city? I mean, you turn into a real slug, face it.

N. I like cities, but that's the trouble—Seattle isn't much of a city. But there are a lot of worse places.

R. It's not a city-city like back East, right? Anyway, we're both going to be here for a couple of years; we've both signed on for next year.

N. You have to let them know in October.

R. Yeah, two weeks after you start, they ask: "Are you going to be here next year?" And you say, "I . . . I . . . am I going to be here the rest of this year? You mean I can stay? You're asking me?" The first few weeks are so scary you think you have more responsibility than ever before, though you probably really don't. You're being watched pretty carefully. You feel like it's all falling on your shoulders and you don't feel you can call anybody to ask for help because you're supposed to know. For God's sake, you're from Alabama, and there's somebody here from Harvard, you're not going to show yourself to be a fool in front of him.

N. And then he found out the real truth about people from Harvard.

R. And I hardly knew anyone when I came to this city, just one person.

N. I knew one person—my wife. No wait, there was someone else, one of the other residents, Judie Kahn.

R. Boy, is she manic.

N. I've known Judie Kahn since college; she used to sit next to me in biology lab and I'll tell you. . . .

R. Boing, boing.

N. She would just freak out in lab—so intense. . . .

R. She just bounces off all the walls: boingg, boingg.

N. There are a lot of angry people in medicine. I know a lot of second-year residents who are really bitter from a combination of things. There's been some inequities in workloads and some people have been taking leaves of absence and not making up the time. People are feeling that the system isn't flexible at all. There isn't a lot of good feeling among the second-year residents; they never coalesced as a group to help each other, and that has resulted in a lot of backbiting—you know, get what you can for yourself and to hell with it if it screws up anybody else. And this attitude just multiplies.

R. There are also a lot of people in pediatrics who don't even like kids, who are just interested in research and are only doing this to pass their boards. I really don't understand the reasoning.

N. Well, if you want to be, say, a pediatric immunologist, it's very hard to be appointed to an academic position if you haven't been boarded in pediatrics.

R. So a lot of people don't want to practice, they are just biding their time here, and some are in the wrong business—they went into it for the wrong reasons, and it's not what they expected at all. But I'm pretty pleased with the year. The city is great; you can get outdoors pretty easily. The best way is when you go out on a transport and pick up a sick baby. The other day, I had to go about fifty miles north, up near Arlington, near the pass, and as we drove I was just sitting there, looking around at all the mountains, watching them all go by from the truck.

N. That's the nicest part. On the drive out you are really encapsulated, no beepers.

R. No beepers.

N. They can't get you.

R. And usually someone pleasant to sit and talk to.

N. Who did you go up with?

R. Donna. Do you know Donna from orthopedics?

N. I probably do by face, anyway.

R. She's the one with the glass eye. But listen, I've got to go.

N. Catch you later.

Nick turned to me.

This day is really incredible; I am basically done with my work for the day. I'm doing a surgery rotation just now, and the workload is variable; it's just pre- and post-operative care, and they're not doing any cutting today and the kids I have are all stable. If I really wanted to I could be doing a lot of the cutting and sewing myself, but it's not something that I'm ever planning to do again.

I don't know what I want to do eventually. I'm thinking seriously about doing three years of pediatrics and then doing a psychiatry residency. Psychiatry is not as demanding timewise, at least during your residency. You see, I haven't been very satisfied with pediatrics; it just isn't what I enjoy doing; it's not what I'm best at. I think I'm best at listening to what patients say and helping them to get in touch with what is bugging them. When I'm feeling energetic, I can say, "Oh yeah, it makes sense to get boarded in pediatrics before psych, because in a hospital setting pediatricians would listen to me more, since there is a tremendous barrier between psychiatry and medicine." But when I'm depressed, I think, Shit . . . two more years of not talking to people.

My biggest frustration with medicine is that I like doing a lot of other things, and medicine really obliterates most of the rest of your life. All I can say is, it better get better later on. I'm very committed to basing my life on something that's fun. And it is hard, because I was raised in the tradition of puritan discipline and delayed gratification, and I've certainly bought into that in a big way. It's a tradeoff. I certainly wouldn't want to live my whole life the way I'm living now. I'm not sure I even want to live three years this way. [laugh] At the end of that time, it is going to change, and I'm going to have more time for other things, and hopefully I'll get more satisfaction out of the work. What's really frustrating is that I get so tired that I can't experience parents' needs, and kids' needs when they are old enough to talk. When I'm this tired, I just don't want to talk with them. I just start seeing that as an added drain that I don't want to have anything to do with, because I want to get home and have some time for myself. The system makes it worse by not giving you any reinforcement for spending any time with the patient; it's not recognized. If you don't write progress notes on your patients every day, somebody will come around; the nurses run around making sure that there is a note on the chart at least every few days. If you don't do a discharge slip, my God, the wrath of God descends on your head; you can literally be put on probation for something like that. And if you don't call the patient's private doctor to let him know what is going on, people get very upset. And obviously if you don't check up on lab values, you are spending money ordering tests, but not checking them out. So there are a lot of things to do that are time consuming, but if you don't do them people will come down on you. Yet you can go for weeks and weeks and never talk to a kid's parents, and nobody will give a damn. This generates a situation where doctors leave all the interpersonal things to the nurses, who usually do a great job, but the doctors have more of an opportunity to help. Patients will open up more to a doctor, because they want answers; they want the anxiety of the situation to be alleviated or resolved. But if the nurses weren't here, I'm sure the kids would all be psychotic. [His beeper sounded and a voice told him to call paging. "Excuse me, I've got to get this page." He left the table, returning minutes later.]

One of the hardest things about being an intern is the pace at which you live, and the work is so focused that it doesn't allow you a chance to step outside and see anything that is happening. It's really weird to see every day the most intense human experiences possible. It gets to be commonplace, it doesn't get integrated, and in some respects it can't or you'd be incapacitated yourself. I end up feeling that it is a strange situation here, but there aren't any chances to step back and make some sense out of how I'm changing as a person, whether the needs I have are getting met, and if they're not, why not and what to do about the rage I feel when I'm overworked, when I feel like there isn't any time for other people, no time for myself—that's hard, you know?

I think there should be an hour a week where every intern gets to talk to their shrink, an hour a week where we don't have to do our work. When I go home, I'm so tired that I don't want to think about what has happened, since that's hard work and I don't want to do any more work. I want to do something mindless, like turning on the TV. But I think doctors would be better in whatever they did— pediatrics, surgery, whatever—if one hour a week there was a time when somebody was going to work with you to understand the experiences you had been going through. But it doesn't happen, because the whole system isn't oriented that way.

As Ray was saying, you're so uptight and anxious about whether you will be able to do the work that it is pretty hard to admit you might be failing. It is hard to start thinking and talking about that. So far this year I haven't felt like I couldn't do the work, but in order to do it, I've had to limit everything else in my life. This year I have spent a hell of a lot of time doing stuff that I fundamentally don't get a lot of satisfaction out of doing; that phone call was about adjusting blood gases on a preemie. A lot of these decisions are not obvious, and they're certainly not "uninteresting because I know it all"— because I don't. The problem is that I don't get satisfaction out of being so organized all the time, getting lab tests, manipulating things, dealing with the technology. After putting in fifty IVs, I can do it, but so what?

Medicine was an ambivalent choice for me. In high school I took physics senior year and I clearly remember thinking, "That's the last time I'll ever use a slide rule in my life—I love English and I love writing, and that's what I'm going to do, that's for sure, that's that." When I got to college, I took organic chemistry as a sophomore and dropped it because I was doing so badly and I said, "That does it,

I'm never going into medicine. I'm not cut out to be a doctor." Then one summer I spent a month as a patient in a hospital recovering from a mountainclimbing accident. I got really turned on by the social milieu, mostly just by lying in bed and listening a lot, and I got on pretty good terms with everybody there. I thought to myself how stimulating and fascinating it would be to work in a hospital. So I went back to school and started to do better . . . and here I am!

The Patient Comes
First, Bingo

WAYNE VAN SICKEL, DIRECTOR OF PEDIATRICS
RESIDENCY

Behind his closed office door, Wayne Van Sickel was confer-
ring with a resident. He was the director of the pediatrics residency
at the prestigious medical center—the residents' ombudsman and
taskmaster. The resident's voice was barely audible. She was a shy
but hardworking woman. Then Van Sickel's reply started up, the
words indistinct but the cadence unmistakable; rhythms of exhorta-
tion, of fatherly encouragement, of humorous instruction. Again he
stopped and was listening.

"All right," he called as the door swung open and a white-coated
woman brushed past. "Let's get this interview started. I've got a
hell of a long day ahead of me yet."

His office was small and filled with the usual journals, file cabinets, and bookcases stacked with textbooks. The dark green desk
was pushed against the wall, so that Van Sickel and I sat face to face,
in close proximity. His ruddy, crew-cut features seemed larger than
life, reflecting the intensity of his presence. He snapped out words,
then bit them off short as a bulldog might (in fact, a stuffed version
of the Yale mascot looked on from the bookshelf). Although he
eventually leaned back in his chair, with arms behind his head as he
scrutinized the ceiling, he seemed all the while to be speaking from
a height—the height of experience, of energy, frustration, and
anger.

I had come to him with the words of Dr. Winn and Dr. Peters still echoing in my head. I was wondering why residency had to be so demanding, whether there was a better way to train physicians. But the first time I talked with Dr. Van Sickel, I got no further than telling him that I was writing a book about what it was like to be a doctor. He was off, firing a barrage of powerful words in my direction.

Two months later, I spoke with him again. It was the same kind of rushed situation, but this time I was able to directly ask the question why residency had to be so hard. Dr. Van Sickel had plenty of words on this subject as well.

Okay, Okay. You want to know what I think about running a training program. I get the message.

Let's start by giving you some background information, and I'll try to give it to you briefly. As a young man I was capable of winning scholarships based on my athletic abilities, and my hope was to become a graduate of either Annapolis or West Point, in the family tradition. But I found out that I was 4F after receiving football injuries and entered medical school intending to go into military medicine, because anyone—regardless of their physical condition—can enter the military medical corps.

I trained in pediatrics because of the experience I could get working with infectious disease. If you look at the history of war you find that up until modern warfare, the outcome of most wars was determined not by skilled excellence of military leaders, but because most of the sick people in the army died, and they ended up with no army. Modern medicine has been a great contributor to recent war efforts, because of its ability to build morale by rehabilitating wounded people. You can get men to go out and shoot at one another and damn near kill themselves if they understand that if they get hurt they've got a 90 percent chance of being brought out and salvaged.

What I found when I entered military medicine as a pediatrician was that it was basically a support service. Caring for the dependents of military personnel meant carrying out repetitive medical procedures so mindless and thoughtless that it drove me crazy. After the five hundredth otitis media and the twenty-fifth meningitis it got to be routine, and I got no kicks out of it. Most of it was acute episodic illness, or self-limiting diseases, or behavioral-management problems which any good grandma could have taken care of.

So I began to seek a career which would challenge my mind with problems which were insoluble, and which would give me an opportunity for an interrelationship with young intellects that were interested in something besides diapers. I had no qualms about not wanting to go into private practice: taking care of stinking little asses of kids that needed to be raised by grandmothers, and participating in the sociological phenomenon of pediatricians pampering rich middle-aged women. I came back to a university setting and began doing research on handicapped children, and running the residency program, and this is what I've been working in ever since. I find that working with the complex problems of childhood chronic disease is a tremendous challenge, and I also get great satisfaction out of dealing with other health professionals: surgeons, physical occupational therapists, and others.

Because of my personal background and my professional feelings, I still put in sixty or eighty hours a week. But I have a very difficult time finding responsible people who feel the same way I do, to help me take care of my patients. By my standards, most practicing physicians and young physicians in training—regardless of what the new youth are saying—are primarily interested in ripping off the public and getting power. Well, I say the patient's welfare comes first, bingo. And if you see a problem it gives you an opportunity to investigate it and follow it through, spend time reading about it, researching the literature, and if you can't find a cure then you develop some method of care.

In the residency program, it's exhilarating to see the brilliance, concern, and conscientious output of the same percent of residents now as there were when I started twenty years ago. On the other hand, twenty years ago I would have one, two, at the most three people whom I would consider avariciously motivated monsters.

My experience is that this group is now five to ten times larger than it used to be—comprising 25 to 30 percent of the trainees. These people are taking advantage of the system, of their colleagues, of the nurses that work with them, and of their patients. Some of them are just peculiar nuts who want to go to medical school and get some kind of a graduate degree because they want to prove they can do it. The system has created a challenge for these people—they go into medicine as "the highest profession."

On the whole, though, the intellectual capability of all the residents today is much higher than it was fifteen or twenty years ago. There's no way that the residents of yesteryear could compete with today's residents. This might be due to the huge number of people who are now applying to medical school, but there's no question in my mind that all of our resident applicants are acceptable intellectually. The only thing that I'm discouraged about is this increased attitude that "the world is for me and it's my apple, buster, and fuck you if you get in my way."

I don't know whether this attitude starts in medical school, or whether medical school selects this type of person. But I've been an assistant scoutmaster for thirteen years, taking the boys into the woods. Before my knees crapped out on me I hiked about 150 miles a year with them. Two of the boys, whom I watched grow up from age twelve or thirteen, were outstanding Eagle Scouts; handled the kids under them perfectly, and they were classic physician material. Both were extremely interested in medical school. I was sort of a role model for them, but they couldn't get in, because they were four- to five-tenths of a grade point too low. Now, there were two other kids whom I saw go from age twelve all the way through medical school. They were both absolutely brilliant, dishonest cheats who took advantage of everybody. They were so nuts that I was afraid of them. Eagle Scout badges were given to them over my protestations, and they got into medical school easily. Well, I wouldn't trust them with the care of a goddam dog.

There're two different philosophies of medical education. One is the Harvard system, where the medical school says, "Since we are made of God, we have therefore selected gods, and therefore the students we accept into the medical school must create ungodlike activity to be kicked out." They put a lot of money into the selection process, and if down the road they realize that they've chosen a loser who is both brilliant and crazy, rather than admit they made a mistake they say, "We'll keep him—we'll cure him." I've had medical students come to me and say they're creating havoc because their family wants them to be doctors, their teachers want them to become doctors, but they don't want to do it! So their family or school sends them to a psychiatrist.

The other philosophy is exemplified by where I went to school. They got all 120 of us together in a room and said, "Something like 95 to 100 of you will graduate, and the rest will scratch."

I feel that both medical schools and residencies should be run with very high standards, and I think that people entering the process should be given the option of leaving if they find their personality is wrong for the environment.

This is part of the purpose of residency training. For four years, students have been puttering around with the science and the art of medicine, without any real responsibility. The only way they can learn to be responsible is by taking care of patients. And the only way they can know if they are cut out for medicine is if they get some practical experience. You want to put residents who are entering clinical-medicine fields under the kinds of stress that they will experience in practice. They find out during the intern year if they want to be real doctors or if they want to become consultants, or program doctors, or something else. If they like that first year, they'll find that an intern works about the same number of hours a year as a physician in private practice. If they don't like it—if they want to spend more time with their wife or something—they should go into a different profession besides clinical pediatrics—they can go into ophthalmology or something.

I think work is good for people. In fact, I work harder than most of my house staff. I've had one day off in the past month. That's because it's my life-style and I like it. Medicine is a service profession, and people who don't like the intern year should get their ass out of medicine. I have no tolerance for that attitude—they're here to serve people, not to make money off of them.

Sure, you can be efficient while you're working thirty-six-hour shifts. I was able to be efficient when I was a resident, and I don't think the physical stamina of our current young generation has deteriorated any. When you get older you can't hack it. If we've got a resident who is over thirty I'm concerned about their physical stamina. But the reason most students and house staff cannot perform is because of their frame of mind. It's exhausting to them because they complain, they're not motivated to work. That's a very difficult concept, which can be boiled down to four letters: L-A-Z-Y.

If you take a look at our good house officers—I have a classic example: she is now a resident in anesthesia, in her sixth year of training. As a senior resident, she was on approximately 120 nights, and she never complained to me once. Some of her fellow residents who were on as few nights as 40 or 50 complained to me constantly: they were overworked, the work was too difficult, they had to go home at ten in the morning because they had been on call the night before. All that was pure, unadulterated horse shit. Barbara is female. She's not anywhere near as tough as I am, or the boys on her service, but she's a good physician. She takes care of her patients.

You see, you have in medicine what's called a team effort. You have two or three doctors on for the night, and they don't go home until the hard work is done. When you have an excessive workload, you give some to another person on your team who is healthy. You don't go home just because it is four-thirty or five o'clock. When I was a house officer and I got tired, my resident would say to me, "You're tired, go to sleep," and I went and slept. The only time we had any difficulty was during a massive polio epidemic when the entire house staff worked as hard as we could, and every eight hours one of us would sleep. I didn't go home for a period of three months, but I got my sleep. I never got overfatigued.

But there's a different attitude now. Everybody has to go off Friday night and Saturday and Sunday, and work not more than eight hours a day. In Europe you see this to an extreme, with socialized medicine restricting monetary rewards for hard-driving, intelligent men. Some of them over there only work two hours a day.

It's very difficult to separate out the motivated from the unmotivated until you work very intensely with them as house officers. I'll sit down with some of them and say, "Look, you've got these kinds of problems, which are keeping you from delivering quality patient care." Instead of their saying "Thank you for the evaluation, because I'm really going to try and improve my performance," they respond with "What kind of an ass hole are you? I'm perfect, and this program's lousy. I'm going to rule you and I'm going to get a lawyer and I'm going to sue you."

These people, when you look at their records, have had straight A's since they entered the educational system. They are good-looking, intelligent people who come in here, and they finally get to the point where it's no longer the system that's giving them grades. They are here to serve the public, and the public is making demands on them. Even though they have no concern for patients or colleagues or anybody else, I can't get them to listen when I say "Look, you are a perfectly good, competent person, but you've gotten into the wrong field." They look upon that as "failing"— therefore I must be wrong, because they've never failed in anything.

Now, I've told you that I got miscast myself when I ended up in military medicine. I told you that was a pain in the ass. But I admitted it to myself very quickly and decided to serve out my responsibility and do a damn good job and then get myself the hell out of there. Even now I get myself into difficult situations as a representative of the residents who are trying to get a fair shake out of the system. The professors at the university want to have resident bodies around to take care of all those midnight problems, because the faculty doesn't want to get up at night. I'm in the middle of all these tremendous pulls. I've gotten into trouble because I use bad language to administrators and I say what I think, but every time I've gotten into trouble has been because I was trying to help my patients and my conscientious house staff. I do this because I have a contract to help them. But I can also say to somebody, "I've had it, I'm not going to have a contract with you anymore. I think you're a jerk, now please blow off." All right?

Residency Years

The hospital stood on the outskirts of Harlem in New York
City, a solid mass of cream-colored stone and concrete. It rose up
amidst ramshackle storefronts, battered apartment houses, and the
lecture halls and offices of Columbia University. On this sticky
August morning, the sun's heat rising from off the wide streets and
glass-littered sidewalks, was already blurring the shapes of shop-
pers, loitering kids, golden taxicabs, and clattering trucks. There
was a chance there'd be showers later in the day.

Beyond the entrance marked EMERGENCY in neon letters, the
waiting room was beginning to fill. A mother rocked her baby,
cooing Spanish syllables. An old black man held a bandage to his
forehead, and a boy stared at the ceiling, his face swollen and dis-
colored.

Beyond the security guard at the entrance to the treatment area,
beyond the "triage" nurse who did the initial screening and filled
out the preliminary forms, Bob Wainwright was getting ready for
work. Dressed in hospital whites, he explained the flow of patients
through the emergency room in a serious yet friendly manner, in
the tone of a person who had given many explanations, many instructions. He pointed out the different rooms opening onto a central hall: the trauma room with full surgical facilities, the orthopedics room with plaster spatters on the walls and ceiling, the
cardiac-emergency room, the obstetrics and gynecology examining
rooms. Bob looked down a long hallway to a closed door. "That's

where the triage nurse sends the psych patients, the crazies, okay? The psychiatrist has lots of potted plants in his room—pretty nice."

He was a senior resident, in his third year of an internal-medicine residency. This night would be his last in a six-week rotation as director of the hospital's emergency room. "When you first find out that residents pretty much run a teaching hospital, it can seem like a lot of responsibility, but there's a certain inertia to a hospital's function. As director of the ER I'm primarily a consultant for the interns and junior residents. Actually, a lot of being a resident is going to meetings. Right now I have to go to Friday-morning ER rounds."

He moved toward a door opening into the main hospital complex, passing in the corridor two patients asleep on gurneys (portable beds). One of them, a woman, had a blood stain running across her scalp. "They're waiting to be X rayed upstairs," Bob explained, "and they're in the hall because we're so short on space."

In the conference room, twenty doctors and nurses shared coffee and doughnuts while some of the week's emergency-room cases were presented. A visiting ob-gyn specialist heard a surgical resident tell of a case where a twisted fallopian tube presented as a pain in the lower right quadrant. Another case of abdominal pain led to a diagnosis of stomach cancer, for this presentation X rays were placed on the wall screen and examined closely by several members of the house staff. There was a lengthy debate about the difference between a tumor and an ulcer on a barium X ray (one on which the patient swallows barium and the X ray records its passage through the digestive system). In the middle of this, Bob had to leave for another conference—morning reports of the medical service. Walking upstairs, he checked a pocket notebook for the names of patients he had recently admitted into the hospital from the emergency room. There were seven from the day before, "and the youngest was seventy-eight years old!"

Morning reports was a smaller gathering—five residents and two attending physicians. There were more coffee and doughnuts, but Bob pulled out a pack of cigarettes instead, as did three or four of his colleagues. Throughout the meeting one felt the stir of nervous activity—fingers tapping on the table, styrofoam coffee cups being dismantled bit by bit, and the inevitable pages ("beepers") going off and a resident leaving the table to make a phone call in the next room.

"All right, let's get started." The chief resident bent forward with an impatient laugh: "Does anybody have any interesting cases?" A dark-skinned resident with darker circles under his eyes spoke up. "Yeah, there was a DKA [diabetic ketoacidosis] who came in last night and died for no particular reason."

The chief resident laughed again, looking from face to face. "Come on, Dr. Santos, that's not very interesting."

"Well," said Dr. Santos, "this patient's son is a doctor, and he was really upset about the way the patient was handled. Things were bonkers on the ward for a while last night."

"Jesus Christ," breathed Bob.

The chief resident had stopped smiling. "Why don't you present that case after we go over the other admissions?" The discussion went around the room, each doctor presenting the patients he had admitted. The doctors recited relevant statistics with ease: blood-urea-nitrogen, serum-sodium levels, sedimentation rate, white-blood-cell count. There was laughter when someone described the vital signs of a 105-year-old patient who had come in for observation. "Nothing wrong with that old guy," one of the attendings said. "I wonder what his secret is?"

Then everyone fell quiet as Dr. Santos described the DKA's death. "It's really a mystery to me," he said. "I know his sugar was out of control for a while in the emergency room, but we got some insulin into him before he was admitted. The acidosis was resolving, when all at once we stepped out of the room for a minute, and he went into respiratory arrest and died."

"Did you say his nucleated-red-blood-cell count was twenty-eight?" Bob asked. "That sounds like CA."

"Yeah," Dr. Santos replied, "beyond doubt the guy had some form of metastatic cancer—his son told us that."

"Have you got the autopsy report back yet?"

"There's not going to be one." Dr. Santos sounded weary. "The son refused to allow an autopsy."

"The bastard," said Bob, "I mean, he should know how important it is to know what his father died of."

The meeting broke up after some talk about the inaccurate blood values reported by the night shift of lab technicians. "If you need an accurate hematocrit at night," advised the attending, "do it yourself." Bob walked back downstairs to the emergency room.

Now the ER was a study in motion—patients, doctors, nurses, and orderlies circulating constantly, filling the air with directives in English and Spanish. A potted geranium beside the ward secretary's typewriter seemed the only stationary living thing. As Bob Wainwright arrived, a white-haired woman was being wheeled into the trauma room. The junior resident, a tall and expressionless woman in her late twenties, asked Bob for assistance. She was trying to put a long plastic tube through the patient's nose and down into her stomach. "No," choked the patient, "no, take it away." The old woman reached for the tube to pull it out. Each time the resident tried to insert the tube, it emerged from the old woman's mouth.

A nurse came in and held down the patient's arms. "Mrs. Simmons, we're trying to help you. Your stomach is bleeding and you need to swallow this tube. Come on, take a drink of water." Her tone was stern.

The resident tried again, while Bob held a cup of water to the·patient's mouth. The tube appeared between the patient's lips, and she spat a stream of water across the nurse's chest. "Take it away!" she repeated.

"Mrs. Simmons," the nurse clenched her jaw, "that was not necessary, to spit on me. Now, if you don't swallow the tube we'll have to put you asleep to do it."

"Let me try," said Bob, taking the tube from the resident, who disappeared into the hall. His voice took on a cooing, fatherly tone. "Mrs. Simmons, you're a very sick person, and we need to stop the bleeding in your stomach. Now please help us by swallowing this tube, won't you?" He inserted the tube in the woman's nose and worked it slowly, keeping up a calming chatter. "You're doing fine, Mrs. Simmons, just fine." At last the tube was in all the way. The nurse put suction on it, and dark particles of blood spilled into a tub. The nurse began to pump ice water down the tube.

Bob left the nurse with the patient and picked up a phone just outside the trauma room. "Hello, is this the medicine ward? How many spare beds do you have? . . . Well, this is Dr. Wainwright in ER. We've got a GI bleeder who's coming up with a lot of coffee grounds. Yeah, we're lavaging her now, and I'd like to admit her as soon as possible."

Nearby, an intern was starting an IV on a man lying in bed in the hall. The intern was having trouble finding a vein, and after several tries his bemused expression disappeared and he put some bandages on the bleeding needlemarks. "This is ridiculous," he was saying under his breath, "I only want to be an ophthalmologist."

An orderly picked up a handful of glass tubes filled with blood. "I've got to run these up to the lab," he said. "I hope I don't miss anything good. You see, I'm doing this every Friday while I study organic chemistry. I'm a pre-med at Columbia. This is fantastic experience, working here, but it really is a war zone—society's war."

The pile of patients' charts at the nursing station grew higher. Bob diagnosed a child with a cold, then went to the next room, where a man was worried about his chest pains. A bilingual nurse helped him explain to the man that such pain was a normal part of recovering from open-heart surgery, which the patient had undergone two weeks before. Stepping out of the room, Bob said, "For a lot of these people on medicare and medicaid, the emergency room is their family physician. We see every problem."

It was well into the afternoon, and Bob had skipped lunch, as usual. Gradually the tide of patients slackened, and Bob had a chance to brief the junior resident about the differential diagnoses of chest pain—how to tell anginal pangs from something serious. The phone kept ringing for him, and he coordinated several more admissions. Another old man, red-faced and bald, lay on his side in the hall, vomiting. The orderly fetched a basin. "I've never done this before," he said.

At six o'clock, Bob went up to the cafeteria for supper. His fiancée, a med student who was working in the hospital's lab for the summer, joined him. "Okay," Bob said. "Now I've got a few minutes to explain how a residency works." His New York accent twisted his thin mouth into a wry smile as he talked.

"Let's say a seventy-year-old woman with congestive heart failure comes to the emergency room," he said, taking a bite of lasagna. "She's sick, okay? Someone evaluates her in the ER, and decides to admit her. That person calls the ward resident—a junior—and tells him that he's getting a patient. The junior tells the intern—there are usually three interns per ward who rotate days—and the intern has to come down to the emergency room and pick up the patient. The intern has to take them upstairs, make sure that all the lab work has been done, find out the results, get the patient to X ray and see that X rays are taken, examine the patient, and formulate a problem list. The problem list includes what kind of things we want to take care of in this hospitalization, what kind of diagnostic workup, what kind of treatment the patient needs, that sort of thing. After all of this, the junior resident comes by and examines the patient, takes another history, and then says to the intern; 'Well, I think you understand the case, now this is what I want you to do,' or maybe, 'You really missed it, and this is what's really going on with the patient.' "
So the intern is supposed to figure everything out, and the junior resident is supposed to make sure that the intern is right. When you're an intern, you think that all this responsibility is riding on your shoulders, but when you become a junior, you realize that you never really had to think during your internship. Someone else was always right behind you, backing you up. When you're a junior, you understand what it means to be responsible for a patient, and then you're responsible for thirty at once, because you're running an entire ward, okay? That's right, the junior resident has three times as many patients as an intern, and there's no one else who is going to say, "That's my patient." There are people who can act as consultants, and there may be an attending who is legally responsible, but . . .

The junior is really a step removed from the patient-care process. He may or may not see a patient every day, depending on how he handles his rounds. Some residents will make only "chart rounds," where they stand outside the patient's room and go over the chart, questioning the intern who presumably has checked over the patient in the hour before. You know: "How is Mr. Jones doing today, do we have his SMA 19 back, what's his potassium or his liver-function test like, why is his bilirubin raised?"

What a residency boils down to is experience, okay? As a third-year medical student you may work up and follow two or three patients each week, so that in a twelve-week medicine residency you may follow thirty patients. If you do a subinternship in your fourth year, you work up six or seven patients a week for six weeks, so there's another forty patients. But when you're an intern and resident, you're seeing patients constantly—several hundred go through the ER in a day—and you begin to get a sense for the spectrum and course of diseases. That's what the differential diagnosis is all about—the sort of discussion that goes on at patient conferences. There's no way to get a differential diagnosis out of a book. You could memorize a few flow charts, but that's all. What a differential diagnosis involves is in-depth experience with a variety of problems.

What happens is that as a junior, you're still learning, but you have also become a teacher and supervisor for the interns. Then as a senior you teach the juniors and help run the hospital. The work doesn't slack off too much right away. Both interns and juniors take call every third night throughout the year. As a senior, I take call only every sixth night, which is nice. But I didn't mind being on call too much—you make a physiological adjustment to it, you really do. I enjoy doing internal medicine. If it wasn't enjoyable I could never have gotten up every day and worked those crazy hours.

The first two years of medical school depressed me. It was anti-intellectual, competitive, and time consuming. Then during my third and fourth years I enjoyed the patient care but didn't feel I had much responsibility, and there was the constant pressure of pleasing my professors—currying a good recommendation. My residency has been a totally different experience. It's been a hell of a lot of fun. After all, I have a provisional license to practice medicine, I'm learning how to be a teacher, and there's something nice about a paycheck arriving each month instead of a student-loan application.

Working in a hospital with this kind of patient population, about half are black, and a third are Spanish-speaking, I've discovered some things about the residents I work with. For one thing, many of them are extremely racist. Say there's a drug addict who probably has endocarditis—most of them do—and who is also black. The resident will refuse to admit him on the grounds that the medical problem isn't that interesting, and anyway he's just a drug addict. I see this all the time, even with residents who consider themselves to be basically liberal. They get overworked and depressed, they get bored, and eventually when they have one more alcoholic with ascites, or one more fat old lady with diabetes who doesn't speak English, and it's two o'clock on a Friday morning, it stops being any fun.

What's more, a lot of the house staff are elitist as hell. They come to this hospital because it has a prestigious reputation. They feel somehow different from and superior to their patients. There's little empathy or identification. The residents want to live an upper-class life-style. Most of the seniors are planning to go into some nice private practice at the end of the year.

Bob Wainwright looked at his watch. "The shifts have changed," he said, "so now I'm running the hospital. The biggest job is finding enough beds for all the admissions. Since the city started closing down hospitals, places like this have been crazy. First, though, I have to go back to the ER to check on a few admissions."

In the hallway of the ER, an old black woman lay on her gurney. Her face was puffed, her lips dry and unnaturally reddish. "She's had chemotherapy for over a year—bad metastatic CA—and now I think she's come in to die. I wish I could admit her and give her a quiet place to sleep, but I'm not sure there's room. I have to save a bed or two for emergencies. Can you hear me, Mrs. Thomas?" The black head nodded slowly. "Mrs. Thomas, how do you feel? Not too well? Would you like a drink of water?" A groan escaped from the chapped lips. Bob found a cup of water, and with a fluid motion cradled Mrs. Thomas's head so that she could sip a few drops. The lips attempted a smile.

In the room across the hall, a woman was screaming. Bob stepped past the dividing curtain and joined an intern and a nurse who were wrestling with a black woman in her forties. The woman's pajamas kept falling down during the struggles, and the nurse replaced them each time. The woman was trying to pull out her tubes and get out of bed. "I can't breathe!" she wailed.

"Let's get her into the trauma room and give her more oxygen," Bob said. "Is she an asthmatic?" The intern nodded. As the nurse wheeled the bed across the hall, the patient grabbed wildly for the nurse's throat. "I'm going to die. Get ready, God!"

Within minutes, the oxygen had calmed her down and she could breathe. "O Lord," she said, "O Lord." Bob leaned over her. "You're going to be just fine," he said. "Try and relax."

The woman sank back on her bed. "O Lord," she said in a singsong, "you've got to help the doctors. They're doing all they can, but they can't do it without your help. You have to show them the way. Oh, Lord."

Several policemen came through the swinging doors, wheeling a stretcher that held a young black man. His face was caked with dried blood. "My legs!" he called out. "Don't touch my legs!"

A policeman followed him into the examining room. "How many hit you? Was it a gang?"

"Oh, there were so many . . . they had pipes . . . I didn't even know them."

A nurse came in and began sponging off his face. The man contorted. "Have you ever had your teeth broken before, honey?" asked the nurse. The man shook his head, and when his mouth opened the jagged fragments of his remaining teeth gleamed.

Another policeman leaned over the nurse. "Would you like any coffee?" he asked.

"Is there a medical doctor anywhere?" someone called. Bob strode down the hall and found a room where a resident was trying to control a writhing, bearded man dressed in filthy blue jeans. "What kind of drugs have you been taking?" shouted the resident.

"Jesus," said Bob, "that's a grand mal seizure."

The man was suddenly still, looking around him. "Where am I?" he asked frantically.

"You're in the emergency room," said Bob. "What kind of drugs have you been taking?"

"Meprobamate . . . lots of them, but I stopped three days ago. Where did you say I was?"

Bob nodded to the resident, and left the room. It was time to make a tour of the hospital, he explained. "I'm going to try and find you a hospital bed," he said to Mrs. Thomas as he walked past her.

His footsteps echoed in the long, high hallways of the hospital. The huge building was sinking into a darkened peace, like a museum after closing hours. The nursing stations on each ward were islands of light.

The night nurses smiled and hissed at Bob as he walked past them. "Sorry," one said, "no room in this ward."

"Thanks," Bob called back cheerily, "but I'll just take a little look myself." By the end of his circuit he had located four empty beds: one in medicine, two in the intensive-care unit, and one in the coronary-care unit.

On the ground floor, he stopped at the entrance to the hospital chapel. Polished wood and brass gave off flecks of light in the dark, spacious chamber. The air was cool near the marble floor. "When this old hospital was built, in the nineteenth century, the architect had many of the patients' rooms opening onto the chapel. He hoped it would help with the healing.

"Look over here," he continued, walking past an ornate staircase left from the original hospital entrance and stopping at a large framed picture on the wall. It was an intricate lithograph in several colors. A lovely Victorian structure nestled against a backdrop of parks, fields, and farmhouses. Carriages were pulled up before the entrance way, their elegant lines dappled with shadows from spreading sycamores. "It's beautiful, isn't it?" said Bob with a reverent tone. Then, after a moment, he announced, "My next chore is to check on EKG's—electrocardiograms—that have been taken today. They're hard to read until you get used to them, so the senior resident on call does a lot of it. The interns have taken the EKGs and are waiting for my confirmation. I haven't formally met all the new interns. They started last month, but by the end of the year we'll be a pretty tight bunch."

Back upstairs, he picked up a heavy chart at a nursing station and detached an EKG from its paper clip. The paper tape was three inches wide and several feet long. Bob moved it through his fingers like a stockbroker checking the tickertape. His gaze darkened. "Dammit, this is no good. There's no base-line measurement." He picked up a phone next to a nurse who was quietly writing. "Hello, could you page Dr. Clark? . . . Hello, this is Dr. Wainwright, I'm SAR tonight, and I can't read your EKG on Dorothy Somers, you forgot to standardize it. Yeah, I know. It's so easy to forget to do it, but I'll have to ask you to repeat the reading in the morning. Thanks an awful lot." He hung up and stretched. "I know it's no fun for that woman intern, who will have a little more work for the morning, but I've got to be honest with her. Oh, I hate this time of night. I start getting irritable and letting little screw-ups like this bother me."

In an alcove off the intensive-care unit, two residents were having coffee and dessert with one of the nurses. There was juice, fruit, and milk in a small refrigerator. Bob stopped in to tell a few stories about the day—the 105-year-old man, the asthmatic who had become psychotic. The talk shifted to vacations. The half-light of illuminated dials and switches showed smiles. One of the residents was planning a sailing weekend for the following month. "I'd invite you, Bob, but this is my one chance to spend some time with a few nonmedical friends."

"How the hell did you stay friends with anyone outside of medicine?" asked the other resident.

The clock on the wall said two. Bob walked to the wing of the hospital, where narrow halls had many doors opening off them, as if a college dormitory had transplanted itself. His on-call room was twenty feet across—"a lot bigger than the one I had last year, but there's no damn air conditioning." But through a dormer window, one could see that it had begun to rain, a soft drumming against the zinc roof. A novel and some shaving gear lay on the bedside table.

Bob sat down on his bed; the mattress sagged almost to the floor. "Well, it's rare enough to be getting any sleep on call—three nights out of four I'm up all night—so I'm going to make the most of it. Good-night."

Downstairs, the ER functioned without him. The beaten boy had gone to X ray. Mrs. Thomas had been admitted to the medicine service. The drug addict was asking for breakfast. "That's fine," muttered the surgery intern, "he can eat breakfast at the same time as the rest of us."

A mother had brought in her baby with a cold. "Can anyone speak Spanish?" called the nurse examining her. A man in another room complained of abdominal pain. "He's hurt for three weeks, but of course he decides to come in now," said the intern, rolling his eyes skyward, "of course, why not, it's only five in the morning!" Minutes later, the intern entered an empty examining room, flopped onto the table, and turned off the light.

Bob Wainwright bent over his breakfast of oatmeal and coffee. His eyelids drooped, and his white uniform was rumpled and bloodstained. A dapper man in his thirties sat down and introduced himself—he was a research fellow in infectious diseases. Bob was beginning a six-week infectious-diseases rotation. Someone else was now running the ER. The research fellow turned the talk to malaria, antibiotics, and the pleasures of working with infectious diseases. "The ER," he said, lingering over the foreign quality of the word, "I don't understand how you guys do that to yourselves."

Part III

Practicing

. . . I will follow that method of treatment which, according to my ability and judgment, I consider for the benefit of my patients, and abstain from whatever is deleterious and mischievous. I will give no deadly medicine to anyone if asked, nor suggest any such counsel; furthermore I will not give to a woman an instrument to produce an abortion.

With purity and holiness I will pass my life and practice my art. I will not cut a person who is suffering from a stone, but will leave this to be done by practitioners of this work. Into whatever houses I enter I will go into them for the benefit of the sick and will abstain from every voluntary act of mischief and corruption; and further from the seduction of females or males, bond or free.

Whatever in connection with my professional practice, or not in connection with it, I may see or hear in the lives of men which ought not to be spoken abroad, I will not divulge, reckoning that all such should be kept secret.

While I continue to keep this oath unviolated may it be granted to me to enjoy life and the practice of the art, respected by all men at all times, but should I trespass and violate this oath, may the reverse be my lot.

—from the Hippocratic Oath

"Sooner or later," the successful psychiatrist told me, "medical training steers almost everyone, no matter what their original intent, down the golden road to practice."

For the medical student dreaming about paying off loans that often total sixty or seventy thousand dollars by the end of residency, and for the resident looking forward to setting his own work schedule, practice seems indeed like a golden road. And whether a physician chooses a solo practice, group practice, or a salaried position with a public-health service, health-maintenance organization, or university, the overwhelming majority of MD's spend most of their time practicing patient care. There is the usual number of restraints: state licensing boards, codes of ethics determined by the state medical societies, the expectations of one's patients and co-workers. But more than ever before in a physician's career, there is an opportunity for personal approaches to the work to develop and be tested.

The six doctors talking about their practices in the following pages look out at the world of practice through the particular prisms of their personal experience. They cannot hope to speak absolutely for the nearly 400,000 medical practitioners in the country, but their motivations are basic human ones. The satisfactions and frustrations they have experienced are universal.

To Have My
Own Patients

RALPH SIMON, PEDIATRICIAN

It is the doctor just crossing the interface between residency training and practice who has the memory of still-vivid first impressions. Often these doctors can point to a single incident, a single patient, or a solitary spoken word that helped them understand exactly how things had changed, how it would be necessary to adjust.

While spending several days with Dr. Ralph Simon, who only months before had begun a pediatrics practice with the U.S. Public Health Service, I was witness to one of those watershed moments.

Dr. Simon was a slender, bespectacled man in his early thirties, who went about his work in a quiet, careful manner. After three years of residency in pediatrics, he had spent one year as a chief resident. This was his first year in actual practice.

Dressed neatly but without the formality of a white coat, Dr. Simon had just finished afternoon rounds, seeing his patients who had been admitted to the hospital. There was a little boy with croup who was amiably carrying on his fight for breath inside a plastic tent kept warm and humid with steam. There was an infant born prematurely who had been gaining so much weight under the care of the neonatal nursery that Dr. Simon had said she would be released to her mother the next day. And there was another child, a tiny girl, who for some reason was not gaining weight at normal speed, her condition labeled with the vague heading "failure to thrive."

Dr. Simon had examined the children, written notes in the

charts, adjusted medications, and conferred with some nurses and residents about each patient. Now we were seated in his small office, sipping afternoon coffee. When the phone on his desk rang, he picked it up and listened briefly before turning to me. "One of my patients, Betsy Ferreira, is waiting with her mother in the outpatient clinic. Let's go over there. Betsy will need some help getting to my office."

He had said the patient's name with a certain uneasiness. On the way to the outpatient clinic—it was not a short walk, although it was on the same floor—Dr. Simon presented Betsy's case.

"She's an eleven-year-old girl with a pontine glioma—a brain tumor pressing on her cerebellum. This is making it difficult for her to balance and move normally. When the tumor was discovered two years ago, it was already well advanced. The neurosurgeons performed exploratory surgery and found a lesion too close to vital brainstem structures to be operable. They biopsied the tumor and closed her back up, and the biopsy revealed a malignancy of a type unlikely to respond to chemotherapy or radiation. Still, a course of radiation therapy was tried two years ago.

"Since that time, the tumor has progressed, and last week Betsy had to leave her old school to begin classes at a special center for disabled children. The expanding mass in her brain has been blocking the normal drainage of cerebrospinal fluid, so she's had several artificial draining procedures—shunts—to relieve the intracranial pressure. The most recent shunt was last week. I became her doctor several months ago, partly at the request of her mother, who wanted someone to talk with Betsy about her prognosis. The surgeons had stayed fairly removed from the case."

Dr. Simon's voice had grown steadily quieter, and he stopped talking altogether as we turned the corner and walked up to the outpatient nursing station. In the waiting area just beyond, a girl and her mother were sunk into one of the low sofas. Betsy was thick-set and apparently asleep, her head covered by a bright blue handkerchief and slumped forward, her eyes heavy-lidded behind thick glasses. But as Dr. Simon walked up, she stiffened and pulled on the arm of her mother, a short and very pregnant woman who had been deep in a magazine. As they stood up together, Betsy tightened her grip on her mother's sleeve, her leg braces clacking together.

Walking back toward Dr. Simon's office, Betsy let her doctor and her mother support her as she shuffled down the long corridors. Little was said. The main sound came from Betsy's braces striking the worn linoleum, the noise punctuating her clumsy movements. As we reached the room, Dr. Simon guided everyone in and arranged chairs in a tight circle so that he could sit facing Betsy and her mother.

It was a simple office with a desk, bulletin board, small bookshelves, and one or two posters on nutrition and health. Above the doorway was the only personal touch—a wide poster showing a panoramic view of snow-covered mountains.

Dr. Simon leaned slightly toward the mother.

"Mrs. Ferreira, how have things with Betsy been going this week?"

The woman sighed. "Oh, better, now that she's started that new school. I talked with some of her teachers, and they seem helpful—they're setting up a special program for her."

"I'm tired," said Betsy in a slow, deep voice.

"Dr. Simon, do you know anything more about her chances? Have you talked with the surgeon about more operations?"

"I spoke with him after the shunt. He said there were no new developments except that the shunt was supposed to ease the pressure on Betsy's brain, helping her with her coordination problems."

"But since last week she's only gotten worse. She's falling down a lot and beginning to wet herself in class. Does this mean that the tumor's getting larger?"

Dr. Simon paused, then spoke slowly. "Yes, as far as anyone knows, it's still progressing."

Betsy's head was drooping again. Her nose had begun to run, a moist glinting under her right nostril. Her kerchief was slightly awry, showing the stubble where her scalp had been shaved for the shunt operation.

Mrs. Ferreira shifted impatiently in her chair, jiggling her swollen belly. "What I mean is, my husband and I both need to know. What is the outlook, Dr. Simon, do you know how long she will live? Will she die this year? next year? We need to make plans!"

A muscle at the corner of Dr. Simon's mouth tightened. Instead of answering he turned his chair to face Betsy more directly. The girl had slid even further down into her seat and was breathing heavily, drooling, on the verge of sleep.

"Betsy?" he asked, his voice rising even as it grew softer. The girl stirred and looked past him, trying to focus on the picture of mountains.

"Dr. Simon," Mrs. Ferreira began again, her tone sharper.

"Betsy," said Dr. Simon, "we've been talking about this brain tumor business. You've heard people say a lot of things about it. Can you tell me something about what these brain tumor things are?"

Betsy was sitting up, watching Dr. Simon's narrow, artist's hands move through the air. He spoke again.

"You know, this stuff is all kind of confusing, but really, what does it all mean? Can you tell me what this brain-tumor junk means to you, Betsy?"

Her guttural laugh cut through the stillness in the small office. She was smiling in an odd, spasmodic way.

"Junk," she repeated.

"It is a lot of junk, isn't it Betsy?"

She nodded.

"Do you know what the words 'brain tumor' mean, Betsy?"

Betsy shook her head vigorously, her eyes lively and excited.

"Well, can you point to your brain, to where your brain is?"

Betsy tapped her head as well as she could with her index finger.

"That's right." Dr. Simon swiveled in his chair and got a pencil and a piece of paper from a drawer in the desk beside him. "Now, watch. I'm going to draw a picture of what we're talking about."

As he drew an outline of a human head in profile, Betsy began rocking frantically from side to side, gripping the arms of her chair, trying to move closer. Her mother and I helped draw her chair up to the desk.

"You see, Betsy, this is a person's skull. The skull is like an outside shell for the brain. Can you show me where the brain is?"

Hunching over the diagram, Betsy again shook her head.

"It lies underneath the skull, filling up this whole area." He motioned to the drawing. Then, glancing across the desk top, he reached for a cylindrical cardboard canister containing modeling clay.

"Here, I'll show you something else." Pulling out a fist-sized lump of clay, he rounded it with a pumping motion of his hand, then showed the empty canister to Betsy.

"This is like your skull," he said, gazing intently at her. "And this"—he held up the clay—"is like your brain. Do you see how it fits inside your skull?" He replaced the clay.

"Uh, huh."

"Now, a tumor"—he looked around again, then picked up a plastic toy car that was resting on its side at one corner of the desk, beyond a copy of *Pediatrics*—"is like this car, trying to fit inside your skull too." As he said this he wedged the front end of the car deep into the clay inside the canister. "But it gets bigger and bigger, and pretty soon there isn't enough room for them both. That's where the problems start, Betsy."

The girl held out her hands, and Dr. Simon gave her the canister.

"Dr. Simon, you still haven't said whether—" Mrs. Ferreira had been left by herself.

"Betsy. . . ." Dr. Simon had not broken his gaze. "Do you understand a little better now?"

Her eyes opened wider, and she moved her lips as if to speak. With one hand she pulled on the car, freeing it from the clay. She turned it several ways for inspection, looked again at the canister, then lunged forward and sent the car whizzing across the table and clattering to the floor. She let out a grunt of satisfaction.

Half an hour later, once the session had been completed and Betsy and her mother escorted back to the clinic, Dr. Simon and I sat talking about what had happened. He seemed deeply affected by the encounter and measured out his words, a few at a time.

Today was the first time that I ever had to directly tell a patient that they had an incurable medical problem. The very first time—and this is after four years of postgraduate training—a full six years of clinical experience! During my residency, if I had to tell someone about a difficult and awful diagnosis, I could defuse it for myself by talking about the hope, by talking about what we doctors could still do for the patient, keeping alive the possibility that through some activity, some more involved procedure, the medical center could offer that patient a chance.

Certainly in this situation I don't want to take away all hope. Pretending that somehow I can definitively predict what is going to happen would be unjustified and inhuman. I would never take away a patient's defenses—the patient will leave them behind when and if he or she wants to. Today I was just trying to bring Betsy to a point where she might want to.

You see, even before today, Betsy wasn't naive. For two years she has lived with the reality that there is something inside of her which is not going away. She knows that the shunt procedures haven't changed it, and that the radiation therapy two years ago didn't change it. So I've watched her perceptions change in the month since she's been my patient. I first used the word "tumor" with her three visits ago, used it a second time two visits ago, and then in preparation for the surgery last week I had talked with her about shunts and what they actually do.

When I talked to Betsy today, I was really surprised that she sat up and became awake all at once. I guess I had assumed she was tired from her organic illness, and I didn't think she had the degree of muscle control to do what she did with the clay and the car. What happened happened because of the groundwork that she and I had established over all the previous visits. The only guidelines I knew to follow were the signs that she was giving me if I could watch her closely enough, be attentive enough to her reactions, so that I could know when it was getting too threatening, or when I had lost her when things got too confusing.

Before I could talk with her about whether or not the tumor was curable, she and I had to find a way of talking about concrete things—what is a tumor, why is it causing trouble—and that's why the clay worked so well. If the whole concept of the tumor had been too new, there would have been a message from her to stop. Every-

thing has to be titrated—all doctors learn the biochemistry of titra-
tion, right? Instead, Betsy was telling me, "Not only do I understand, but I already know, and I can say the next step," which to me
translated into "I will allow you to say the next step."

Now that I've shared the truth with Betsy it feels better . . . no, it
feels awful at the same time. It makes me admit some of my own
frailty, puts me in a position where I might lose control, and I don't
want to start crying in front of Betsy. I've worried about that.
There's all the frustration of not being able to cure someone who is
so young, at not being able to cure the world with all the medicine
I've been taught, finding the difficulties of not getting the desired
end result, having a sense for what my patients are going through,
but at the same time coming to know my limitations.

It's been hard to stay with Betsy since her prognosis became so
grim, and now it's hard to face the future, to experience the next few
years with her and her parents. I know that even now, no matter
what I say, Betsy and her parents still have some fantasies that I
possess some hidden magic, that I can make it all go away. I'm tempering those fantasies a bit, but they're still there. What's more, the
parents are still tremendously guilt ridden about how they never
suspected there was a tumor until it was too late. And now they're
wondering how emotionally attached to her they can become, since
they know they're going to lose her.

All of this—this staying around to listen to the reverberations of a
patient illness, discovering the consequences to Betsy and her
family—it all feels new. It's been the big difference between residency and practice—to have my own patients, to follow them
through, even when I can't cure them.

While I was working as a resident in a tertiary-care medical center, the patients seemed much more naive. Even if they had leukemia, when they came to the hospital to be diagnosed they would be
thinking that here is one more disease that the doctors can magically
cure, since the doctors fixed my strep throat before, they fixed my
pneumonia before. And if I had to share bad news with them as a
resident, I would be too busy to stay around to feel the aftershocks,
to find out whether the way I communicated with them was as effec-

tive as I thought it was, or whether it was inadequate. We have a built-in defense mechanism as physicians—perhaps all professionals have this—that allows us to fill in a gap in our knowledge with self-assurance. As a resident in this kind of situation, the gap would be "I really don't know how well that bad news sat with my patient, but since I haven't seen him again, well, things must be going okay—I would have heard if they hadn't!"

So, starting practice is really a big and very lonely responsibility. Before, I was a part of a great and very powerful training institution which provided tertiary care. Much of this specialized, high-level care involved making up for the mistakes and having the final say over the misdiagnoses of the L.M.D.s—the local medical doctors. As a resident I had a tremendous security in being able to turn to both other residents and specialists—the clinical professors who can offer not only extra experience and knowledge but also the ability to allay physician anxieties.

Now that I'm stripped of this incredible support system, I see why so many doctors find it hard to really listen to patients. It's because they're still carrying on a dialogue with themselves to convince themselves that they can be competent in a scary medical world, fighting with the need to know everything, to come up with right answers. Here I am in the same position as all mistake makers are in. Now I'm an L.M.D., and I've found that the primary physician is put in the position of dealing with fewer diagnostic findings with each case, encountering earlier, more equivocal signs, and having to live with the present uncertainty and the ensuing months of uncertainty.

But then there's that feeling that I've had with Betsy of really communicating with a patient, of building the rapport, the trust, finding out whether what I'm saying is getting through, and to be learning how to share with Betsy the feelings of "you know, it really is awful and frustrating to be dying, not to be able to run like the other kids, not to be able to talk the way you want to talk." And then listening to her responses, and saying back to her that her questions are not dumb, that her illness is something we can talk about. I'm learning a lot of lessons I never had as a resident.

I Wanted to
Touch People

DAVID GOMEZ, FAMILY DOCTOR

The word physician still brings to mind the image of a solo practitioner, although the number of doctors making it alone has declined in recent years. In solo practice, there is no intermediary between the doctor and the clientele. The doctor's reputation is a delicate construction upon which both doctor and patient must rely.

How does one establish oneself in private practice? How does one learn to walk the fine professional lines of the doctor-patient relationship? And if one lives in a small community, how does one draw distinctions between friends, neighbors, and patients?

Again trusting first impressions as touchstones, I found in a small New Mexican town a doctor who was willing to answer these questions. It was Dr. David Gomez' second year of practice in family medicine, and he had already honed to a fine degree his awareness of the place in the community that he was beginning to fill.

Dr. David Gomez also wove several other threads into his story— how it feels to become a doctor against the odds of poverty, racial discrimination, and physical frailty. He was also unusual for returning to practice primary-care medicine in the region of his childhood, resisting the lure of lucrative urban practices or a prestigious academic career. His life and practice are based on choice, and tempering that choice is a strong sense of heritage and an almost instinctive sense of the need for someone to do the work he is doing.

Toward the end of a Sunday afternoon, David Gomez was saying good-bye to the members of his family—father, mother, sister, and nephew—who had come visiting from their small town thirty miles away. As they walked toward their car, the relatives' faces shone in the long rays of the July sun—faces as brown as the New Mexican scrub, which stretched away over the ridge behind David's house, and wearing a look of pride. David Gomez had become a family practitioner in the New Mexican town of Las Cruces; and his comfortable home and the Datsun 240Z in the driveway testified to the same thing: that he had succeeded. Only the nephew seemed unimpressed. The young boy was more interested in the horned lizard scuttling about in the cardboard shoebox that he carried under his arm.

David stood in the doorway and watched them drive off. He looked young for someone beginning his second year of practice, his blue-black hair combed back neatly, his thick black glasses giving a scholarly look to his angular, smooth-skinned face. With a smile he showed me into the living room and took a seat in a comfortable chair. In the next room one could see a pool table, more furniture, and the entrance to a modern kitchen. Later in the evening he would point to these material possessions with a laugh, saying, "People come here sometimes and say, 'Look at all the expensive things.' I say 'Yeah, but I'm up to here in hock for all of them.'" Then he would laugh, in the special way he had of combining notions of success, misfortune, and humor.

His life in medicine had consisted of just this combination. He joked about how young he looked for his twenty-nine years. "When I was working at the student health clinic two years ago, a woman came in for a Pap test, and when she saw I was going to do it she freaked out. Maybe the fact that I was Chicano had something to do with it, I don't know. She said I was too young to be a doctor. She said, 'How do I know you're not just some weirdo putting on a white coat?' Right then I said, 'Forget it, I'm not going to examine this lady—if she can't trust me, she can go somewhere else.' That's the only time that ever happened."

We talked late into the night, sipping beers. Tomorrow morning would be the start of another six-day work week, but Dr. Gomez plunged into conversation with freshness and honesty, putting fatigue aside in his eagerness to share the story of his practice. His enthusiasm made it seem that his family extended far beyond the visitors who had left and the wife and children asleep in the house. It also included the community that he served.

He was quick to point out the need for objectivity in the way he approached his work. "I won't treat my wife or my children, and even though my nurse sometimes asks about something, I can't treat her either. I tell her, 'Charlotte, you're one of the family now.'" But even though he could distinguish between his immediate family and the immense variety of people who came to his office in ever greater numbers, the sense of closeness and familiarity prevailed as the night wore on. Several times he had to answer the phone, prescribing warm-water enemas for one of his hospitalized patients, getting the EKG results from another, checking the antibiotics dosages for a third. "Talking on the phone becomes a reflex," he told me after one of his trips to the kitchen. "I just pick up the receiver, and even if it's the middle of the night, something in my mind shifts into gear and says 'Medicine.' Most of the time the problems aren't monumental, and I don't like to have any other doctor taking my calls. I'd rather be the one taking the calls on my own patients; that way I never lose control over what is going on."

When I asked him how he started along the road to becoming a doctor, he leaned his head back and laughed. "Well, for one thing, nobody knocked on my door and handed me an M.D. degree."

It's a long story. I grew up in a small town about twenty-five miles south of here. My parents never said to me, "You've got to become a doctor." There was never much support for it. When I was three and a half I had an operation for a congenital hip dislocation. Even with the operation I've had to use crutches and a cane a lot, even now, sometimes. So when I would go in to see the doctor about my hip, he would say, "David, when you go to high school, work hard, because you really need to think about going to college. You ought to get a sit-down job—have you thought about being an accountant?" Now, as time went on, I became interested in science, studied it a lot in high school, and my parents said "Look, become a pharmacist, they work good hours, and, yeah, they don't get paid that much, but you get to sit down on a stool." In the back of my head, though, I knew I would rather be a doctor than a pharmacist. I didn't want to push pills, I wanted to interact, I wanted to touch people, I wanted to help them.

My high school had a graduating class of twenty-seven people, and somewhere along the line I got messed up trying to get college scholarships. The head of the school board had a son who was class salutatorian, and he got all kinds of nice scholarships. Well, I came in highest in my class—valedictorian—and I got a fifty-dollars-per-semester scholarship to the University of Texas. That was back in 1968—we were a little dumber then. My sister said, "Look, you don't have to go to Texas, you can go to New Mexico State." And when I called New Mexico State they checked my financial status. My dad's a barber and doesn't make much, and they said, "Oh, yeah, we can give you a loan." So I ended up at New Mexico State here in Las Cruces.

In my first year of school I was a chemistry major, and I had some ideas about going to medical school. Everyone I talked to said, "Forget it—you're the wrong color, you're not going to get in, your dad's not a doctor, you're handicapped, you're not going to get in. Study something that you can do after four years, okay?" Yeah, I was really encouraged [laughs] but I talked to this friend of mine whose mother was a Chicana. His father was an Anglo, and he said, "Do you really want to get in? I'll show you the ropes." He went and got all the literature on medical school, how to apply, and he said, "Don't pay attention to those other guys. You've got the grades, now just go ahead and try it." So I ended up applying to U. of Texas, and Harvard, Washington in St. Louis, and University of New Mexico as a last resort. I got interviewed at San Antonio and at UNM. I could have been interviewed at Ft. Worth, but I didn't have enough money to get up there. But I got in at Houston and Ft. Worth, and San Antonio, and at UNM. I could have gone anywhere! All these people who had warned me were really surprised—a lot of them who did better than me in school didn't get in anywhere but UNM. That's when I realized that nobody should have tried to discourage me. I was upset . . . discouraged, I don't know.

When I got to UNM I met Atencio. He's the one in the administration who pulls for the Chicanos. There was a problem a few years back where qualified Chicano students would apply and their applications would get lost, so that when the admissions committee would meet to say yes or no on a candidate, they wouldn't have anything to discuss, and the student would be put into the "maybe" file. When Atencio got there, he started Xeroxing everything, so that if the meeting came and someone said, "Oh, we haven't got the file on Gomez," Atencio could say, "Well, I just happen to have the file here." So thanks to him they couldn't get away with it anymore. Now, for me it wasn't a matter of special pull, getting into UNM. I got in other places without any pull. I was qualified, and they took me.

So I did the four years at UNM. I had some problems. At the beginning of my third year, I had a total hip-replacement operation. The week before the operation I went to a doctor for a routine physical, and he told me that my retinas were on the brink of detaching. For this they put me in as an emergency. I had a bilateral retinal repair the next day, and a week after that I had my total hip. It was crazy—they put me in the hospital, everybody knew I was there, okay? I was there three weeks, and I had no phone messages, no visitors from the medical school—zero. The only doctor who dropped by to see me was an osteopath in training! Nobody else came up to say, "Hey, Dave, you're doing fine, sorry to hear you're in the hospital." Nothing, zero, *nada,* zilch, you know what I mean? I was out of the hospital on December 24—it was the worst Christmas vacation I ever had.

For seven days, I had to lie there with my head sandbagged so that the retinas could heal, and with a pin in my hip from the other operation. I was sick in a heavy way. For a while I was even hallucinating—I couldn't have taken that for very long. My parents came up to Albuquerque and said, "Come home, you need rest, you need a break." My grandma came up and told me, "Hey, you've been through a lot, but you're not Superman, why are you so hard on yourself?" But something was telling me: "You're not going to give up, you're not going to quit school, you can do it."

If you've never been a patient, if you've never been there, it's hard to know. . . . I can look at a baseball pitcher and imagine what he feels like, but I'll never really have that feeling of pitching out there and having people watch and cheer. But I've been a patient so many times. . . .

When I was beginning my internship in internal medicine, we were talking over a patient in conference, and the head honcho, Dr. Murphy, asked how many of us had ever used a bedpan. I was the only doctor who had! How can you tell somebody, "Well, we're going to keep you in the hospital for six weeks; you're going to have an IV, but no bathroom privileges; you have to use the bedpan." If you haven't been there you can say that and then go home and have dinner and watch TV, and go back the next day; but your patients, they can't go home.

A month after my hip operation I had my first rotation, in radiology. I was on crutches and anemic—my hematocrit dropped to thirty from a normal of forty-five. By the end of each day I was exhausted—almost passed out a couple of times. But I was going to do it, come hell or high water. After that I did my regular rotations—pediatrics, medicine, surgery, the whole kit and kaboodle. I was hobbling around on two canes, and my pediatrics resident wrote in his report that I "lacked initiative." [Laugh]

All during med school I said that I wanted to come back here to Las Cruces, it would just be a matter of time. A lot of my classmates ended up in California, a few moved back East, and I don't think many wanted to go back to their hometowns. This is a poor state; who wants to stay where it's poor? There aren't the medical resources here, the research centers, the fancy machines; it's not very classy. Some of my old classmates come down here and say, "My god, you don't have this, and you don't have that." Well, I wish we were better-equipped, but I have to make do with what exists in the community. The other guys can go to Harvard and become brilliant cardiologists or thoracic surgeons, but some of us have to be general practitioners, somebody's got to fill the gaps. If they don't do it, somebody's got to!

Only one or two out of fifty have become G.P.s—the rest have gone into some sort of training: internal medicine, radiology. Those of us in family practice are looked upon as flunkies. Even the people who started out from small towns like I did, they got to the big city and Jesus, they'd seen the other side, why go back? A friend of mine was down here visiting. Today is the first day of his fourth year in ob-gyn, and he never fails to remind me how he has continued on while I have given up.

Oh, I could have done it; I could have adapted, become a specialist with the nicely draped office, paneled, and the pretty receptionist, the tables with *Business Week.* I'd come in wearing my tie and a certain type of hairdo. It's not me but I could do it. Matter of fact, when I finished my internship in Phoenix, I was thinking about staying there. I talked to some people in a group practice, but they really wanted someone older who would fit the group, who would play golf on Wednesday, bridge club on Thursday afternoon—the country-club routine. I don't play bridge, or golf, and I'm not into racquetball or tennis. It disappoints a lot of people.

But for my wife and me, our family ties were too strong. My wife's from a town not far from here, twenty miles out on old Highway 28. Her mother's had a couple of MI's, [myocardial infarctions] and there was no one else nearby. My wife liked Phoenix and Albuquerque—the shopping centers, the entertainment—but she didn't want to go away and leave her mother all alone, so she wanted to come back, and she didn't have to talk me into it!

I came down here and started working at the student health center for New Mexico State, but I couldn't make ends meet with what they paid me. The football coaches were making a lot more than I was. So a friend of mine who was working at an emergency room in El Paso heard about two guys leaving a practice here in town and asked me if I wanted to take over their place with him. Well, on April the first, 1978, we started practicing.

We started off easy. A lot of people didn't want to try us out right away. It wasn't like the old days where you bought a practice and you bought both the equipment and the goodwill that the old doctor had built up in the community. All we got was the equipment from two examining rooms, along with some desks and typewriters. The patient records of the old doctor were kept in the old office, and people could just come pick them up and take them to their new doctor.

We didn't starve. I think I made my overhead the first month—not bad. There was a tremendous flux in the patients. I started to lose the Anglo patients to other doctors in town, but I began to take new patients from an osteopath in town whose roster was predominantly Mexican American. We were taking welfare patients, and most of the other doctors in town weren't.

After the first month, I was making my overhead plus. I didn't depend on referrals from other docs, because nobody refers to a general practitioner. My referrals are patient to patient—an aunt to an uncle, to a cousin to a daughter to a son. I see somebody from a new family, and before I know it, I've got that family, and their friends, and their friends' friends, and their cousins, and on and on. My practice has just steadily climbed. The first summer was slow, and people told me, "Well, summer's slow, wait till the winter, it will pick up, and then people will drop you again the next spring." Well, since about the first week of November right through this last Saturday, yesterday, I've had about four days where I wasn't very busy. I'm busy every day, and I'm still taking new patients. If I'm this busy in July, can you imagine December and January?

Most patients, when they check out a new doctor, if they like him, will say, "He's not a bad guy, but before I decide on him I'm going to look at someone else." So they'll check you out. I saw someone last week who had first come in on May 19, 1978. A year and a month later, he's back, and I thought I'd lost him, but no, he just wasn't ill. When they're back, they're back because they have a problem.

I have a few people from Columbus, which is about ninety miles away, people from Hatch, Silver City, Anthony, Deming, Canutillo. If they're from those small towns—Deming or Silver City—when they're sick they don't trust the doctors in Deming, they want to go to the big time. So they come to Las Cruces. If they're from Las Cruces, it's more of the steppingstone thing—they want to go to a doctor in El Paso. And some come to see me all the way from Mexico, when they have relatives in town who want them seen by an American doctor. It makes me feel good that the family brings them past El Paso to be seen by me, their family doctor. They've got to have some faith, some confidence in me.

Whenever I go make rounds, or go to the office to see patients, I'm just myself, I'm in my own environment. My practice is predominantly Mexican American, predominantly medicaid. I know my people, and to them the only thing different about me is that I've had some education. I'm serving a purpose, and I can work with them. There's no problem. Imagine me trying to work with the Navajos. It would be awkward trying to remember how to say "Where does it hurt?" in Navajo, or remembering not to look at the Navajo ladies when I talk with them—to look at them and not down at the ground is a sign of disrespect. So I don't have to worry about those things.

When I go into an examining room and shake an old man's hand, instead of saying, "Buenos Dias, Mr. So-and-So," I'll say, "Que tal"—you know, "How goes it?" And the older people—most would like the doctor to joke with them. I'll have my checklist and be going over the history of present illness. I'll say, "Y su salud, como esta generalamente, ha esta operado, ha esta en l'hospital?" I'll go "Toma alcol?"—do you drink; "Fuma?"—do you smoke; and then "Toma consejos?" which is like a joke in Spanish: do you take advice? And often when I first say hello, I'll say, "Como le va,"—how goes it, "Entre muertos y heridos . . ?" and I don't have to finish, the old guy will know it and get a kick out of seeing that I know it. It's a saying: *Entre muertos y heridos, estamos todos bien podridos*—all of us are basically between the dead and the dying, we're all in that manner, shape, or form. Sometimes I'll say to an old Chicana, "Que tal, senora?" and she'll reply, "Oh poos, entre verde y seco," you know, somewhere between green, live, and dry, dead, and she's like a tree saying to me that she wants to grow more toward the green, can I be of some help? When they see I understand [laughs] that does it—

they realize, hey, he's human, he knows about us, he's part of what's going on here.

Sometimes when I'm working with people who speak only Spanish I get frustrated with some of my medical terms. Instead of saying "red blood cell" I have to say "corpusculo coluntura," and by the time I get it out, it's almost too late, because I never used those words. I learned medicine in English, and as a kid I had to learn all my medical terms in English in case I went to an Anglo doctor. As a kid I would say "la knee," or "su chest," but I can't say that to an old Mexican woman, it has to be "la rodilla," "su pecho." I have to just relax, let the brain say it right, forget about my higher cortical centers.

If a doctor came down here without knowing Spanish he'd have a hard time. If he was really aggressive, he could do it. There's a surgeon in town, Dr. Wilbee, who's fluent. He's from an Ivy League school—has all kinds of pennants from college around his house, but he goes all out. You can tell from the way he works. When he sees a patient for the first time, he's a gringo, but when Dr. Wilbee starts talking Spanish you can see all of a sudden a smile come over the patient, a look of relief, like "Wow, I can talk to this guy." If you're old and Chicano, you want to talk to someone who knows your lingo, it's as simple as that.

The National Health Service Corps was set up to get doctors down to places like this, but they don't care about getting long-term doctors, or getting doctors who will really fit in. They have bureaucrats in Washington that look at a map, and have quotas for how many doctors are needed for what counties, and which are areas of physician shortage. I went through med school on a National Health Service Corps scholarship, because this was an area of physician shortage, and I wanted to come back here. But when I finally left my internship and came down here, I called them up and said, "Hey, I'm moving down to Las Cruces," and they said, "Well, last month we came up with the new figures, and Las Cruces is no longer a physician-shortage area; therefore you have to go to—" and they gave me some other counties. So that's a hassle I'm going through now. My practice probably draws from some of the counties they wanted me to move to, but they don't care. It's sort of crazy. They say, "We've got these many patients, and X number of doctors, meaning X number of doctor-patient interactions, this much equipment, so much for this, so much for that, okay, let's put it in, shake it up, and we've solved the problem, right?" It just doesn't work that way; you can't just throw around money and requirements. When I think about the possibility of national health insurance in the future, I think of that bumper sticker—have you seen it around? It goes "If you like the postal system, you'll love national health care." That's the only thing that comes to my mind.

I really don't know where this business of coming back started. I can't pin it down, I can't give you a cock-and-bull story about when it was instilled. I didn't have to say to myself, "Well, I'm going to be the savior and go out there and convert all these heathens to Christianity." I mean, there is no way I'm going to save these people, and I'll be the first one to tell you that some of the worst people around are these people I'm trying to help. But dammit, if I don't do it, nobody else is going to, and they're either too dumb or too blind to realize it. So help me, I'm going to hang in there and do it for them. Eventually, it will sink in [laughs].

They come in late, they don't keep their appointments, they're the rudest with the receptionist, they can be rude and obnoxious with me. To them it's not that I'm doing something for them when I say yes I will accept your medicaid, yes I'll lose money and time by seeing you, but I'm doing it because I want to. They don't understand that. They expect me to say how pleased I am that they are here, that they have chosen me as their physician. They are demanding—they use their medicaid card like a major credit card for absolutely minor things. "Little Jonny hurt his finger about three months ago, and I am so worried." Boom, there's an office visit right there. Or they come in with a sore throat, or a cold, something that chicken soup would take care of.

Then there are good ones, the ones that I don't mind taking care of, like the person who comes in diabetic and hypertensive because he's obese, and he can't speak English. Some of the people like that, especially the older ones, will treat me with a certain amount of respect—they say, "Oh, thank you very much, doctor." They will like me. With some of them you could even say that they love me, and they make me feel very good. It's becoming a thing of the past in the Chicano community, it's being lost, but for the people about fifty and over, anybody who has education and a position in the community is deserving of respect. The greatest token of respect that one Chicano can show another is to add the letters "Mr." to a person's name. So a lot of the older ones don't call me doctor, they say *Mr.* Gomez. It's like they have elevated me with this title, put me in a position of respect.

It was all part of the background they were raised under. My dad, the way he was taught and the way he taught me was that you're supposed to respect and honor certain things, just like you weren't supposed to show fear, or pain, and as a man you run the house and become the breadwinner. You don't depend on the wife for support—if you aren't the man in the household, you're worthless.

A lot of respect for the elders has been lost now. It used to be a disgrace if a son ever put a grandparent in a nursing home. You just didn't say, "Hey, Granddaddy, you're getting old and you're becoming a pain in the ass; therefore I'm going to take you out to the Villa Manor and dump you there and come see you once a month." You just didn't do that.

When my grandfather was alive, he was one of those tough old guys. He died at the age of seventy-one of prostatic cancer. The first time he ever saw a doctor was when he became obstructed at age sixty-nine. He had never in his life seen a physician—no immunizations, nothing, zero. When he saw his first one, it was too late to do anything. He was the head of the family, you know what I mean? Whenever somebody wanted to buy a car they'd ask grandpa for his opinion, his judgment. We didn't just go out and do something and say, "Hey, this is what I did."

He died in '66, so that he never knew I was going to be a doctor. It's a shame, he would have been very proud. Of course he would have been prouder of my sister, who is a teacher. He had the most respect for *profesoras*—teachers—and after that came veterinarians. He had farms and ranches, and animals, and grew cot-

ton, and anybody who could take care of animals was very important, because without animals the family didn't eat. But he would
have been proud to see his grandson get all this education, that I
took this much time. Knowledge was valued, wisdom was considered a tremendous gift, and he had it.

My parents used to say that whenever their doctor didn't look
good or didn't dress well they felt ashamed somehow, because it was
their doctor and the community had a certain impression of him.
That sort of philosophy is still around with my patients. They want
to see the doctor busy, they want to see him doing well, but they
don't want him to be ostentatious. If they walk into their doctor's office and it's full of people in the waiting room, they say goddam, this
doctor's busy, therefore he must be good, therefore I'm seeing the
right doctor. When they come to my waiting room and it's full, what
they don't realize is that I'm slower than most. [Laughs]

This applies to a lot of things. My house here is in the Tellshore
area, and when people hear that they go "Tellshore; only the rich
people live in Tellshore." But if you go even higher up the slope,
this hillside becomes Imperial Ridge, and if you live on Imperial
Ridge, ah, that's something different. Dr. Wilbee's up there, Dr.
Kesselman, and some of the big businessmen. When we moved
here and bought this house, we could have had a house that is off to
the left of our backyard, we can see it from here, and that's on the
Imperial Ridge. We went up to look at it, and I said no. There was
something just a little too ostentatious about it. You know?

The other day I was shopping for a new car, and I really wanted to
get a nice one, a Riviera. I didn't know if we could even afford it
after I paid my taxes, but I took it out for a drive and started thinking, do I really want to be seen in town with this? Right now I drive
my Z, and people say, "Oh, the doctor, he's as crazy as the rest of
them, drives a sports car." But if I got this new car, they would go,
"Did you hear what the doctor's driving—a Riviera!" Somehow that
would stick in the craw of a lot of my patients. They would go,
"Geez, look what he does with my money, and he charges so
much." But if they come in and see that I'm busy, it's different. If I
come in late they'll say "Yeah, banker's hours," but I tell them "No,

I went to the hospital this morning and made rounds. If you were in the hospital, I would already have seen you." That kind of knocks them back, and they realize that I've already been out there since seven-thirty in the morning.

You have to do a little bit for your patients, you know? My partner, my ex-partner, I could tell you about that—about people who are into medicine for other purposes. He used to whip through thirty patients in about two hours or so. When you do that to a lot of people, a lot of them are going to be dissatisfied. My partner started out with a bigger practice than I had, and by December he was only seeing six or eight people a day. He had to go moonlighting in the El Paso emergency room to make ends meet. Plus he always would come in with his boots caked with mud, never wore a tie, always wore jeans, and he lost patients because of his approach. Some people who came to see him said, "I don't want to be seen by a doctor who comes in smelling like horse sweat in the morning, I don't want to be seen by a cowboy or a hippie." My partner was real cool, he would act like "Man, I'm doing my thing, I'm dressed like a cowboy, and I'm not at all part of the establishment." Well, great, fine, but his patients weren't tolerating him.

I don't wear my tie everyday, because sometimes in the summer I just can't take it with the heat. I wear my white coat in the office, but all my coats have a little patch sewn on. One has a Tweety Bird, one has a roadrunner, one is Sylvester the Cat, and there's a Speedy Gonzales. My patients will see my white coat, and then they'll see the little patch—the Tweety Bird. It's only for the kids, and the white coat is for the older patients to show them that I'm not coming in without my white coat on, sterile and all.

Have you ever sat in a doctor's waiting room waiting to see him? You start to notice things. So in my office there is something which sends out the smell of Kool-Aid, so that instead of the smell of alcohol the office smells like roses or something. To me it smells like Kool-Aid.

I didn't have to have a designer come in to give me ideas about decorating the office. I knew I wanted to have posters up. Some of them are just for fun, and some of them are charts of anatomy.

When they see the anatomy charts my patients sometimes go, "What's that?" but after a while they say, "You mean this is my gallbladder, this is where my pain is happening?"

I try not to make the rooms seem cold. You know the paper on the examining table? I bought paper that has flowers on it, and instead of those white patient gowns, I bought blue ones. And then my nurse. I just ask her to wear something white—doesn't matter whether it's white pants or white shirt, and she doesn't have to wear a cap. It's just formal enough, do you see what I mean? And just a matter of saying yes, I want you to respect my nurse, just as I respect you as a patient.

When I was growing up in Anthony, there was a really good doctor, a family practitioner, who had moved there from El Paso. He's still down there—a very quiet, very, very intelligent, brilliant man, and he's out there in the sticks. If you ever look at his house you can see that it is swamped with magazines and books, all the stuff that he reads. In fact he's got two houses. He had to move out of one because the stuff he'd read and saved had filled up all the rooms. He reads all the medical literature, and also about electronics, geology—they even offered him a place at the university in the geology department. I remember once I got sick and got put on Beta Par, one of the steroids that no one uses very much. I showed it to an internist in El Paso who didn't know what it was, and then when I was down in Anthony and mentioned it to this doctor, he said, "Oh, yeah, Beta Par," and he started rattling off all these facts that he'd read about it. My god, I was really impressed. [Laughs]

He practices a different kind of medicine out there. He has no lab, doesn't draw blood, doesn't take urine. He moves on a lot of intuition, saying, "If it looks like you have a strep throat, I'm going to treat it as such, or if it looks like you have appendicitis, I'm going to send you to a surgeon in town." Mostly he'll say, "It's probably nothing much; here, why don't you take these vitamins and see me if you're not better in a few weeks?" Sure enough, most of the time you feel better.

The way I was trained, I just can't do that. If somebody comes to see me with malaise—just doesn't feel good, a bit of weight loss but nothing else—I'll say, "Okay, let's get the SMA, let's get the 'lytes, the blood calcium, the sed rate, the urinalysis, and the chest X ray, okay?" Especially with medical-legal worries, I don't want to hear "You should have," because it's my butt out there on the line. Sometimes it is to hell with the patient's expense. I'll let them pay their ten bucks for the blood count, and if it comes back fine that's great, that's really nice! And if it doesn't, well, there will be something that I can do for them. The whole malpractice situation scares the heck out of me.

Sometimes I get so discouraged and think Jesus, this is not for me, this is crazy, Uncle Sam is taking me for a ride with taxes and the welfare system. I work pretty hard to make ends meet. I was really busy this winter—one time I had twelve people in the hospital at one time. It doesn't sound like much, but when you make rounds every day of the week and have office hours all week and Saturday mornings too, you get so tired. So sometimes I want to do something with less hours, because I can only do so much, and the leg can only take so much. I can't go out and work in the ER for a certain amount of extra money. I'd like to but I physically can't. I even thought about applying to law school. Sure, it would only be three more years of school, and it would give me a lot of opportunities. But I would lose a lot that way. With a law degree and a medical degree you go work for a big corporation or you go around setting up HMO's, you become an administrator, you get a nice salary, wear a nice suit; you fly a lot of places and you have a nice office. But you lose the direct contact with patients.

That's why I could never be a radiologist, even though it's an easier life. You see X rays all day long, and spend the rest of the time talking to a stupid microphone. I would be a nervous wreck doing that. In Albuquerque there was one resident in radiology who got a call to go upstairs and see a patient and he said, "Oh no, where's my ten-foot pole?" [Laughs] He said, "The next time I touch a patient it will be with a ten-foot pole."

Right now about 60 to 75 percent of my patients are Spanish-speaking, and most of them get either medicaid or medicare, but I see everything from migratory farm workers who just recently came from south of the border to two of the four bank presidents in Las Cruces. I've got university professors, people who taught me bio-chemistry as a freshman at New Mexico State. What's neat is know-ing that I know something they don't, because in college, even after four years, no matter how much I knew they always knew more. Now they can't say, "Tell me about the $1S2$, $2S2$ bonding orbitals." [Laughs] I'll be talking to them about medical things, and some-times I'll be talking to them the way I'd talk to another doctor, and shoo, it will go over their heads. I won't realize it until they say, "Dave, could you explain that in layman's terms?" And then I'll remember that there is something that I know which is special, and even though I have so much respect for my old professors, they are not all-knowing.

I have a few lawyers for patients, and many policemen. I'm sup-posed to be the prisoners' doctor for the city, and I do the physicals for the police department, and I'm the doctor for one of the bus companies. You name it.

For my friends who are going into internal medicine, this week will be their first week out of training. The ones I've talked to have been so excited about being internists, but they are going to miss so much. Have they ever been down in the nursery and had a C sec-tion handed to them, this kid that is seconds out of the womb, because they are the pediatrician for that baby and it's up to them to take care of it? Or to have to go up and take care of the ninety-six-year-old lady who fractured her hip, or seen a four-year-old with otitis media? Or consoled the husband whose wife just left him? Or . . . I could keep on going! They are not going to do that as intern-ists. Yes, it's nice to know so much medicine, and to get a lot of re-spect, and it's true that here in town the family doctors don't have admitting privileges to the hospital ICU. We have to get a patient admitted by an internist.

But I can't see myself going back for two years of training, then coming back here and all of a sudden giving up all of my patients who are younger than eighteen. I mean some of the internists in town will not even do a pelvic exam!

In my practice, the mother will walk in with two of her kids. I'll take care of one for a routine check, and the other one might have an infection, and then I'll do a routine physical on the mother and do a pelvic exam. I'll have done it all—I am that family's doctor. It's a tremendous feeling. With some families I've treated father, mother, sons, and daughters, and then some of the grandparents, I see the whole spectrum. You can go through a family-practice residency now and become a family practitioner, but that does not necessarily make you a family doctor. Do you see what I mean? You can hang degrees up on the wall and impress your patients, or you can talk with other doctors and give twelve differentials for ascites, okay, great, you're a big hot shot, I'm proud of you, you know a lot. But if people who come to you don't like you, if you don't take care of their family, if they don't want you for their doctor, don't care for you, you are not their family doctor.

David Gomez yawned. Monday morning was not far away, the start of another week. "I've had two weeks off during my internship, and four days this Memorial Day, and that's been it. I'm due for another break some time, but I don't like the idea of having some other doctor cover my practice for a while. That's why I'm on call for myself every day. Now, I'll probably wake up tomorrow morning, come into the clinic, and think, 'God, another patient,' but as soon as I see my first one, boom, that feeling is gone."

You're Supposed to Help People

JUDY CAMPBELL, SUBURBAN PEDIATRICIAN

David Gomez' humor plays off the precarious balance between the physician's high ideals and physical and emotional stamina, and the seemingly unlimited supply of needy patients, especially among the poor. The medical needs are obviously one effect of bad housing, malnutrition, bad working conditions—the many facets of poverty. The physician and other health workers often feel the burden of this diffuse need; and what sort of medicine can cure poverty and despair?

Intrinsic to this balance is the capacity for imbalance, the tendency of an idealistic person to take on too much, to "overload." Dr. Judy Campbell is one doctor who reached very high before finding she had to draw back. After a residency in pediatrics she worked at a high-volume clinic serving low-income families and their children in the central city where she lives. When the continuous exhaustion and discouragement became too much for this exceptionally sensitive physician, she left the clinic and joined a group practice in the suburbs. In the two years since the move, she has been able to find time for her new marriage, her new children. She does not regret her choice, but neither has she forgotten the questions her experience has raised. How does one struggle against overwhelming feelings of hopelessness? how does one keep one's ideals and remain intact as a person with a life outside of medicine? And what does it mean, anyway, to say that one wants "to help people"?

"An uncomfortable doctrine," Albert Schweitzer wrote in *Civilization and Ethics*, "prompts me in whispered words: You are happy, it says. Therefore you are called to give up much. Whatever you have received more than others in health, in talents, in ability, in success, in a pleasant childhood, in harmonious conditions of home life, all this you must not take to yourself as a matter of course. You must pay a price for it. You must render in return an unusually great sacrifice of your life for other life. The voice of the true ethic is dangerous for the happy when they have the courage to listen to it."

Judy Campbell paused for a moment to look out the picture window of her study. Through the trees, two small blond-haired boys could be seen walking down a road with a middle-aged man. They were Judy's husband and young sons. "I still haven't found it," she said at last, "that state of being totally happy in my work as a pediatrician. I feel there is more I should be doing, even though I know that there will always be more to do. But these days I'm working part-time to be with my sons and my husband, and that feels right somehow. In many ways the most rewarding times of my life have been with my family, in the last few years."

Downstairs, a teapot began to whistle. "Would you like some tea?" Judy asked. It was a rainy Sunday afternoon, and the big, modern house in a suburb of Atlanta, Georgia, was warm and quiet. Judy busied herself with the tea making, her long, delicate hands seeming to enjoy activity.

Sitting again in a chair in her study, she began to talk about her life as a doctor. She was in her late thirties, but her features were youthful beneath pulled-back blond hair. Her words often seemed a soft-spoken confrontation with herself—halting, wondering, honest. A pained look would cross her face as she blamed herself aloud for the comfort of her suburban practice. The feelings of guilt and helplessness that she expressed seemed familiar to her: she had clearly questioned herself in the past.

At one point in our conversation, her two-year-old son wandered into the room, slightly damp from his walk. Without pausing, Judy lifted the boy to her lap in the unconscious gesture of motherhood. As she did so, the pained expression left her face.

I guess you could say I have a classical, typical pediatrics practice. I see kids for school physicals; I see sick kids and try to make them well, or tell the mother that if they wait long enough the kids will get well by themselves, and I hope to recognize serious illness.

There's a simplicity to working with middle-class families. The children come in and they're not being buffeted or overwhelmed with developmental problems, or marital disputes, or malnutrition. They come in, and they're hurting, and their mothers listen to what advice I can give them. If I say that I'd like them to return in several weeks, they come back on schedule and they've thought about things, they've tried the treatments I may have suggested. It's just—it's an awesome experience to see things move so smoothly. But you know, a few years ago I was working as a salaried employee for an inner-city clinic, and now is the first time that I've worked fee-for-service. I'm very uncomfortable with that. The money that I have to charge appalls me.

I'm in a group practice, and have arranged with the other partners to work part-time so that I have more time for my children. It's wonderful to be able to work part-time, but I also give up a little freedom to work in a group. There's a peer pressure to charge a minimum amount for each patient visit. My partners tell me that we all have to bring in enough to pay the overhead, the secretary. But it doesn't always seem fair. Late last Friday afternoon a mother called me, very upset about the way her daughter was coughing. I agreed to see them at five-thirty, and sent them a bill for a regular office visit. My partners chided me. They said I had to charge that mother half again as much since it was "after hours."

My job now takes a lot less out of me than when I was working downtown. When calls come over the phone, the parents are able to describe their child's condition accurately, so that the sick kids I see are appropriate—they *should* be in a doctor's office. So, I can give advice over the phone, and this will reassure the parents, so that I can usually avoid seeing basically healthy kids after hours. Considering the after-hours rates that I have to charge now, this is the best arrangement.

You know, it's interesting, the difference between fee-for-service and prepaid care. One of my old clinic patients moved out here, and she was used to getting all of this incredible health care free. When I treated her child, the woman ended up being faced with some big medical bills, and she was very angry at me, though she never admitted it. All of a sudden, I realized that I had lost sight of my initial idea of charging people what they could afford to pay.

Why is it so hard to hold on to ideals in medicine?

I come from a Quaker family, and all of us grew up with the idea that we had to "help people." It was just that simple and idealistic. I have a brother and he became a social worker; it wasn't really what he wanted to do, but it was difficult for him to break away from it, to go back to school in history, which was his first love. It was just, you know, a way in which all of us could live most easily with ourselves, if we were "helping people."

After my first year of college, I went to Mexico for eight weeks of work-camp experience with the American Friends Service Committee. Down there I saw this sort of physical suffering that really affected me. I felt I couldn't do much for these people, that I had no skills. I felt very helpless.

Just before my senior year in college my parents sent me off to a vocational psychologist, who did a lot of testing, and I really think he was a frustrated physician who wanted to go to medical school. I never would have thought of going if he hadn't really pushed me. I told him I thought I could be a nurse or a teacher, and he said no, you've got to have control over your own life, you don't want to be doing what other people say you need to do, you want to be doing what you want to do. Now, frankly, that didn't appeal much, but the trip to Mexico had left me with some idealistic images about my life, and so I went into medicine.

I remember I had an adviser in college who said if you apply to medical school you won't get in, and if you get in, you won't make it through. It was as if I had his words in the back of my head the whole time I was in medical school. I was so caught up in the need to be competent that on every test and with every new skill I learned, I was frightened. I remember that working up patients was difficult, and I was feeling awed and a little guilty because this was the essence of medicine, and I wasn't enjoying it. One of the first patients I ever had was a surgery patient who had just been admitted. See, I was at school in Washington, D.C., which is really a southern city, and they had wards full of poor patients, which were all black wards. And this poor black man was obviously really uncomfortable, and here I was trying to get this admission history and physical. He began to get more and more uncomfortable and he was still so polite and courteous, and it went on, and he began to sweat and so forth. I was so incredibly inexperienced that I just didn't know what I was looking at. He had a cardiac arrest and died as I was interviewing him. It turned out later that he had an esophageal carcinoma which had perforated into his aorta and he'd bled out. It was something else, to think of that guy. I guess what gets me the most is my blundering perseverance in the face of the fact that this man was dying, that and the way he maintained his incredible courtesy.

Still, it was the human relationships that kept me going. Once when I was a medical student I happened to walk through the emergency room. I don't think I belonged there at the time; I don't know why I was there. I just walked through and I heard this child screaming. And I don't know what made me do it, but I walked into the little alcove where the child was being seen. It was probably a child about seven, she was having a spinal tap and she was just terrified and she was screaming, the way a rabbit would scream at its imminent death. I walked in and I can't remember what I said; I think I took her hand and told her that the worst thing about the tap was her fear, and she stopped crying and held still and we did the tap. The resident looked up and said, "Thank God you walked in."

I can tell you, there have been a lot of times since then when I've told kids that the worst thing about a procedure is the fear, and it hasn't worked like that. It was just one of those experiences where you do something and you don't know why you do it, and it's sort of awesome, and you walk out feeling funny, you know?

Then there was a patient that I got to know during my fourth year of medical school. He was up on a private floor—a man of about thirty-five with leukemia. When I first walked into the room and in-

troduced myself, he said, "What's your first name?" I thought,
Jesus, what is this? Well, he started calling me Judy right from the
beginning, and it was one of the most unusual relationships I have
ever had. I followed him through and he died during my internship.
Often, when I was done with my work, maybe at ten or eleven
o'clock at night, I'd go up and wake him up and we'd sit smoking cigarettes and talking. He was one of the few people I've seen who was
truly unafraid of dying. He'd say, "I'm not afraid, it's just the me-
chanics of dying that bother me." I watched him get sicker and
sicker, and once I saw him deny it. He wanted to buy lots of new
clothes, even though it didn't look like he would be able to ever use
them. Once he cried, because he wondered what would happen to a
family he'd been helping, some children and so forth. But I remember him telling me that only his wife loved him enough to let
him go. Everybody else wanted to keep him. Right then, I could see
that I didn't love him enough—I didn't want him to die, I was so
fond of him.

One day I came up, and I knew he was going to die that night. I
watched him slip into a coma. He started saying that he was going
on a long trip, and he needed a pilot for his plane. Then he started
talking about building a tower in the sky, way up into the infinite
regions. Finally he died, and I was holding on to his toe, watching
him. Soon I had the most horrible headache, and later I cried because I hadn't been able to let him go, I hadn't loved him enough.

See, if you remember, my motive was to "help people." If you
plan to go out and help people you tend not to look at what needs to
be done but at what you think needs to be done. You can really miss
the boat. You can get too involved because you have this inner drive
telling you you're supposed to "help people," even if you have to
sacrifice yourself, which leads to no end of making a lot of mistakes
and handling things inappropriately. My clinical training, especially
during my internship, showed me sides of myself that made me feel
really bad. Much of it was a matter of survival. I was on call every
other night. There was a sort of fatigue that changed my whole
perspective on the world. I lost track of seasons, I'd go to sleep on

dates. That fatigue never left, and I forgot what it was like not to have this horrendous feeling hanging over me.

We had a very, very busy inner-city emergency room, and I got so coarse, I can remember a woman who came in the middle of the night and she had a bladder infection. She was uncomfortable, but I was so angry at this woman because I had to get up or maybe I hadn't gone to bed that I really blasted her with my anger, and she left without getting treatment. I felt so bad and so guilty. I can think of a couple other times when similar things happened, especially if I was very tired or very hungry and could see myself missing sleep or a meal. I became animal-like, and it's very difficult to have to face that in yourself.

My training gave me a lot of half-skills, and when I got out, I still didn't know where my limits were. I didn't know when to accept the fact that I couldn't do something to change such-and-such a situation. The worst thing was the business of thinking that what I could supply people, because I was "helping people," was in their best interest, when it may not have been at all, when what it was designed to do was quiet my own feelings of guilt about not helping enough. I still was idealistic, and so I went to work for a year at an inner-city adolescent clinic, and after that for four years at another low-income clinic.

When I was working at these clinics, mothers would frequently call me up in the middle of the night or late, late in the evening. They would want to have their child seen, they wouldn't be happy with a discussion over the phone. So, I made a lot of trips downtown, and it took a lot out of me, because it involved an hour of driving just to see one patient. It was all because I either couldn't evaluate the situation over the phone from the mother's description, or else the mother was at her wits' end for some reason or other and wanted to have her child seen regardless of my evaluation. Usually, the child was a lot sicker over the phone than in the examining room.

Then during regular hours, the overuse at the clinic got to me. What I call overuse is a lot of visits from kids with self-limiting viral infections that I couldn't help at all. The mother would say, "This kid is sick, do something for him." In my suburban practice, the mother always has some valid concern—I almost never see a kid for just a cold. The mother will be worried about pneumonia, or ear infections, or something worse.

At the same time, the sickest kids I've ever seen in pediatrics, and I guess you could say also the sickest kids psychiatrically, were patients in the low-income clinic. On my mind is a Samoan child. We had a tremendous heterogeneity of the population there—gypsies and Filipinos and Orientals—an incredibly rich experience to work with people from these cultural backgrounds. This one Samoan child had more problems than any child I'd ever seen. She had a condition I'd never heard of before, an exotic infection. The infection involved her urinary tract as well as her digestive tract, and so she was septic, obstructed, she was on hyperalimentation—it was incredible. I think we had ten specialists in at one time or another, and I was trying to find someone to take the patient over, because I don't feel like an intensive-care physician.

The child's Samoan parents were there, and they had real doubts about what we were doing to their daughter. They watched her get sicker and sicker in the hospital. The child also become psychotic twice—once a manic psychosis on steroids, and once a depressive psychosis. The mother began asking to take her back to Samoa, but we all felt she would die if that was done.

Finally we compromised. The family got some medicine from Samoa, and they brought in some of the high priests, who went through a series of incantations. I was able to watch all sorts of magic rituals. In situations like that I felt I was useful. I kept the parents from taking the child out of the hospital, and gradually she got better.

So I was trying to remain human, to provide humane care. I mean, I got very attached to many of my patients. And I was learning how to use ancillary services and coordinate care. My problem before had been some sort of shyness or lack of assertiveness; it had been hard for me to pick up the phone and call people. At the inner-city clinic I got used to calling school officials, public-health officials, consultants, and so forth. This was a good thing, because after I had been working at the inner-city clinic for a very short time, I saw that I was not enough by myself.

For one thing, I don't work too fast, and the clinic was a fairly high-volume treatment center. Everything seemed so chaotic that it was hard to figure out what the appointment schedule was. I'd be working at my usual speed, and by the afternoon there would be a pretty long wait to see me. In my group practice now I'm working hard to eliminate that sort of thing, but I'm also a lot more aware of how to avoid the problem now.

I just felt like a failure so much of the time. I had the feeling that if I gave a little more, I could be more effective. Finally, I gave up on giving a little more—I just couldn't make it.

I left the clinic and joined a group practice not far from my house. My sons were born, and I began working part-time to be with them. Now I've been out here two years. I miss my clinic families, the youngsters that I watched grow, often from neonates. I hate starting over, but in this middle- and upper-class practice the problems I have to deal with are things that I can get a handle on and maybe be of some use. I feel more comfortable and less helpless about my work now than ever before, but now my Quakerism comes back. I feel guilty even saying that.

The Lucrative Art

Alex Bissel, Surgeon

Dr. Judy Campbell returned again and again to the association of money with medicine. She felt uneasy charging her patients. And in an economy based on freedom of choice, it seems perverse to become rich off the anxieties and infirmities—indeed, the choicelessness—of sick people.

Certainly medical practice is deeply entwined with the world of finance. The average physician currently earns in excess of 70,000 dollars a year—a very substantial baseline. The financial security and material comfort it implies jar with the meager salaries of the residency years, or the huge loans taken out during medical school. Many physicians told me that the lucrative incomes of practice were necessary to compensate for the years of training and education, but why create such rags-to-riches patterns? As one radiologist told me (radiology being one of the most lucrative specialties), "Whenever I was unhappy in medical school, I figured it was because I didn't have enough money. I thought if only I could have enough to pay the bills, everything would be all right. Maybe it was because money was the obvious thing missing from my life as a student and a resident, keeping me from feeling totally satisfied as a person."

Above all, the image of the doctor as enterprising businessman jars badly with that of the doctor as altrustic healer. And in fact, for doctors to be reaching the upper financial classes in such large numbers is a recent phenomenon in the history of medicine. At the turn of the century, there were more physicians per capita in this country than today. This was before Flexner helped cut back the number of medical graduates, saying that economic considerations should be overlooked in the interest of controlling quality. As a result of this glut of doctors, physicians' salaries were modest by today's standards.

The expanding economy and the growing willingness of the federal government to subsidize health care have been kind developments for the medical profession. But growing consumer unrest over doctors' fees and the huge amount of money spent by the nation on medical care each year (currently more than 8 percent of the Gross National Product) has been a key factor in the erosion of the public image of physicians.

What truth is there to the image of the doctor as profiteer? It was a difficult stereotype to investigate. Many physicians talked for hours about their practices, providing infinite detail about the medical care they furnished and never mentioning fees without my questioning. So, I decided to ask a doctor to speak specifically about the financial side of his practice, and of how he reconciled money and medicine in his own life. I wanted to talk to a very successful physician, one who had made a decision to build and maintain a lucrative practice, earning not seventy but two or three hundred thousand dollars.

In leafing through the pages of *Medical Economics*—the medical equivalent of the *Wall Street Journal*—I discovered that the average income figures for physicians are inflated because so many physicians invest heavily with the capital derived from their practices. But while I was in New York, I had the opportunity to meet a physician who based his impressive salary almost entirely on his practice. As I prepared to meet Dr. Alex Bissel, the images of charlatanism ran through my mind. He had agreed over the phone to talk about the money he made, and I was unsure exactly what to expect. But in my hours of talking with this intelligent and articulate man, I discovered nothing as simple as charlatanism.

Base qualities of character exist in everyone, and as long as the American economic and legal climate allows doctors to set up high-volume "medicaid mills" and "diet clinics" and the other possible medical swindles, the descendants of snake-oil salesmen will continue to exist and prosper. So it was more informative for me to meet a physician at the opposite extreme, a striver after an unusual sort of perfection. Dr. Bissel embodied shrewdness combined with a Harvard-educated gentility, and compulsiveness matched with a need to excel in the very lucrative medical environment of Manhattan, where physicians' fees are the highest in the country, despite the fact that there are also more physicians per capita there than anywhere else, with the possible exception of Los Angeles. He was a true practitioner of "the lucrative art."

It took me three tries to be able to talk to Alex Bissel. The first time, he suggested a lunch meeting at his private club just off New York's Fifth Avenue. But his morning surgery—a simple hernia operation—turned into a four-hour effort to remove a strangulated section of intestine. A week later, we planned another lunch, but a woman who had swallowed lye in Atlanta was flown up to New York for Dr. Bissel—a recognized master of gastrointestinal surgery—to operate on. He spent all day dismantling and restoring the ravaged digestive plumbing of the failed suicide.

Two days later was his afternoon off, and he strode through the plush lobby of his club. "Alex Bissel," he said, shaking hands in mid-stride toward the elevators. "Let's go upstairs and find a table."

Most of the diners had finished the main portion of their meals, and the long, high-ceilinged room filled slowly with the smoke of after-luncheon cigars. A huge smorgasbord was in the center of the room, manned by several uniformed waiters. "Oh, good," said Dr. Bissel, walking up to it, "I love a buffet—I always want one of everything."

He was middle-aged but still intensely agile in his movements through a room. His small eyes surveyed his surroundings carefully from behind conservative wire-rim glasses. His stocky frame suggested a lifetime tension between material comfort and physical exertion.

He was happy to talk about his work and what it was worth in financial, medical, and personal terms.

I like to run my own show. I like to be responsible for my own decisions and I like to feel that I have certain superior abilities that will be recognized in open competition. I'm very competitive. I play a lot of athletics; I try to—I *do* win prizes in squash and tennis all over the city. As a team-sport, medal-oriented competitor, I like to win, and surgery is a field where you can win the big one, where you can save a patient's life each time. There's a drama and a physical contact with the patient that is almost unique in medicine.

It's a matter of not quitting. There are a lot of obstacles to getting where I've gotten to, some of which are paper tigers and some of which are real. You have to spend the energy and time to find out which obstacles are real and which can be hurdled or circled. It's a matter of pursuing various paths and restarting when one proves to be unfruitful.

When I finished my residency twenty years ago, the traditional course was to apprentice to a senior surgeon who needed your hours and youth. In return for your coverage of his practice, he would provide you with some office space, and there was the additional benefit of the surgeon's reputation rubbing off on you to some degree for the inevitable day when you were pushed out in the cold.

These jobs were ardently sought-after, even though the yield for the junior surgeon was questionable. I apprenticed with one of the doyens of New York surgery, whose name is still famous. He founded three surgical-specialty boards and more or less invented esophageal surgery, which is my specialty today. I was working for a master, but at the same time I maintained some teaching responsibilities at the hospital where I had trained. When the master died, I was given an assistant professorship at the hospital—a voluntary position, which is very hard to get because the hospitals, in the interest of "protecting their nest," do not like to give out clinical appointments. They prefer full-time appointments, where the surgeon is working directly for them.

When the old man died, I had to scramble for office space. A very kindly medical man with a big office let me have a small space with low rent for the first year or two that I spent on my own, a physician doesn't need a whole office when he's starting. I leased larger and larger quarters over the next ten or fifteen years, until finally, when I became fully booked and was operating almost every day at different hours, requiring a full schedule of follow-up and emergency visits, I opened my own office. This is expensive, but it gives me a latitude that is not available in any other way. I can set my own hours, I have my own help, responsible only to me, and I miss hardly any calls.

If you are successful in private practice, the financial rewards are those of a tennis star who comes in second rather than tenth. There is a geometric increase in your earning capacity as you become able and sought-after by your colleagues. Surgery is still paid for on a piecework basis in private practice, and the minimum wage for a certain surgery has to be at a sufficient level that the neophyte with an occasional case can still survive. If the surgeon is doing three or four cases a week, he's making a good living on the order of twenty thousand dollars a year. If he starts doing eight cases a week, he'll be making forty or fifty thousand a year, and if he does twelve cases a week, he'll be making a hundred thousand a year. There's quite a difference. Having more patients requires more time, but usually the work is concentrated at a single hospital, so that it's not impractical for a successful surgeon to expand his practice. There is a diluting factor when the busy surgeon takes on assistants or associates to handle the volume. There's a limit to what an individual artist can turn out, and of course the work of the school of Renoir is not the same as the work of the Old Master himself. This is where the business of surgery transcends the value of a big surgical practice, and the emphasis falls on treating as many patients as possible. I resent this approach. It denigrates the calling to which I aspire, and it's not the way I like to treat patients.

I like to see patients on a one-to-one basis. The patient is sent to me, and he's my patient. He's not going to another doctor next week and a third doctor the week after that. Because they come to me on a one-to-one basis, they become very jealous of my time. They feel that in addition to the operation I owe tham something in terms of surveillance and meticulous care, which is true. They require my constant ability to be there in an emergency. Practicing as a private surgeon, now that the public is waking up to the fact that surgeons are not gods but people responsible for occasional negligence, can be both interesting and aggravating!

But I don't see anything wrong with making money. After all, the surgeon is responsible for all the suffering, injury, and even death if the surgery is performed incorrectly. The art of surgery makes it a service more valuable than that of the plumber, to my thinking, and even though plumbers are paid excessively in our society, I think surgeons should be paid more. I think that a patient actually respects the doctor who works for a reasonably high fee. He feels he's got a better doctor working for him. No patient has actually said that, but they act like that. Some of my most unpleasant, unhappy patients have come to me on a third-party, insurance-set basis. They've thought of me as part of the plan rather than as their doctor, and both abuse my services and don't appreciate their coverage plan.

A doctor is a leader; he's not in the status of an employee. He is by the nature of his profession someone who makes the basic decision, and the commodity is the patient's health. If you are sick, you don't want anybody but the top man, whoever he may be, making the basic decision about your health. This is a fact that the public fails to understand. They keep saying, "Well, we hate doctors but we love our doctor." Well, by God, your doctor is the man who keeps you from going under during a decisive period, and he is worth every penny to you that he costs at that time. He is your crisis person. I'm not talking about the routine bloodletting that goes on, or the annual checkup complete with the patting on the head— those are more in the commercial area. The business of surgery is in the hernias and the gallbladders and the breast biopsies, which can be done efficiently and routinely with little pre- or postoperative care. The satisfaction of surgery comes from the complex cases. I still have to fight for hospital time and for the best cases, but I'm at a level in my practice where it is challenging to me. I'm a surgeon who operates on people who are either going to die or be crippled if I don't intervene. You're coming to me as a decision maker.

The classic story is the story of Steinmetz, who was asked personally by Henry Ford to come to the River Rouge plant and decide where to position the basic switches for the electrical system of the whole plant. Mr. Steinmetz said, "Do you really want me?" And

Ford said yes, so Steinmetz went to the River Rouge plant and paced the length of it, looked over the whole situation, then took a pencil from his pocket and marked an X at a certain point on the wall. A week later, Mr. Ford got a bill for fifty thousand dollars and was furious. He called up Steinmetz and said, "You're billing me $50,000 for making an X on the wall of the River Rouge plant?" Mr. Steinmetz said, "Mr. Ford, for making the X on the wall of your plant: five dollars. For knowing where to put the X: $49,995. Thank you very much." And Ford paid the bill.

He pushed back his chair. Coffee had been served and we had drunk it. "Let's walk over to my office," he offered. "I want to show you a few things."

On the way out of the dining room, Dr. Bissel paused to sign his club number on the luncheon check. No money exchanged hands. We walked out of the air-conditioned lobby and into the sodden New York summer afternoon, then minutes later entered an elegant steel-and-glass building overlooking Central Park. He climbed carpeted stairs and unlocked a heavy walnut door, which opened into a plush, modern waiting room. Dr. Bissel walked past the receptionist's desk—he had given his nurse and receptionist the afternoon off—and began searching through the file cabinets full of patient records. "Take a look at this bill," he said eagerly, unselfconsciously, handing me one. It read:

Preliminary Examination and Diagnostic Tests:	$60.00
Surgical Expenses:	$4,400.00
Total:	$4,460.00

"You see," he explained, "I work everything into the surgical fee." That includes follow-up visits, hospital visits, prescription fees, phone consultations, and so on."

I charge by the amount of care involved on a case. In determining the exact fee for a certain operation I am helped by guidelines from insurance companies, which are put out to guarantee that they will pay for certain procedures. It's pretty much what the market will allow. Of course I'll tear up my fees for a comrade who says "Take this case for nothing," and if he says "Take this medicaid case," I'll do it. This kind of courtesy is a matter of political expedience. I take one patient for free, and the doctor who sent the patient will next time send the old lady on Park Avenue with the toenail that has to come off, which is worth its weight in diamonds. It all balances out.

For a lady with an esophageal reconstruction and six operations after an intensive lye burn of the esophagus and the pharynx, my surgical fees alone will amount to fifteen or twenty thousand dollars. The weeks she spends in the hospital will cost the government in excess of $100,000. Incidentally, the major costs of illness are never the physician; they are the hospital and the nursing services. But either way, it's a lot of time and money.

Don't forget that I practice in New York, and my overhead is astronomical. I now pay 16,000 a year for malpractice insurance. My office rent runs 15,000, my girls run 30,000 between the two of them, my telephone bill is 300 a month, my office overhead is another 5,000 a year. Above the entertainment part of it, my car costs a minimum of 5,000 a year, what with maintaining it and paying for parking in my building, in the hospital—you can't park for free in New York. In other words, I have to earn in excess of 1,500 a week to pay my overhead. Now, patients don't like to pay that kind of money, and if I did only a couple of operations a week, I would have to have an average fee of five hundred dollars an operation. I have a house in Westchester County and a family to support, with four children who go to school, and this means that I have to be bringing home quite a bit of money after paying my overhead. I'm now grossing two or three hundred thousand a year, which has been pretty steady for the past ten years.

I'm talking about the income for a full-service doctor. I don't have any real free times when my practice slacks off, I'm always busy. I leave the house five mornings a week at a quarter to seven, and I get home between nine-thirty and eleven-thirty most evenings. Most of my time is spent in the hospital making rounds, operating, teaching, making rounds again, with about an hour off sometime in the afternoon where I get to play squash or tennis. I also make it a rule to go in either Saturday or Sunday to check my patients—and this is in addition to the usual telephone contacts with residents or associates, so that routinely I put in a five-and-one-half-day week, twelve hours a day, not counting emergencies. Since there are always one or two emergencies in a week, I put in roughly a seventy-hour work week, average.

I don't derive too much income from consultations, and my office visits are worked into the cost of an operation, so I operate on a tight schedule. Because of the politics of cities and hospitals, hospital beds are constantly being limited in New York. There's a crunch to maintain 100 percent occupancy. I can't bring a patient in whenever I want. I have to wait, always running the risk that the patient could get irritated and go away to another surgeon outside the city who's got an empty hospital. You can also lose patients because you get them in and you can't operate on them because the OR schedule is crowded. There's a lot of static and overlay. And then there is the fact that there are very tight binds over what hospital I can practice in. The hospital is jealous of your time, and if you cannot donate enough time to your hospital, they won't grant you operating privileges. Therefore you're limited in the doctors who will refer to you. They have to be in your hospital group. It's a closed system.

And behind everything is the fact that in New York there is constant competition for cases. If I'm not available to handle an emergency, Doctors X, Y, and Z are. I don't really have to have an associate for when I'm not feeling well—the city takes care of it. There are always four or five surgeons who would be delighted if I said to them, "Hey, Joe, while I'm away, or I'm not feeling well, would you mind covering the phone?" They'll do it, and they'll charge me for it.

One of the telephone lights on the receptionist's pearl gray console had begun to wink. "I'll take that in my office," Dr. Bissel said.

He walked swiftly past three small examining rooms equipped simply with examining tables and equipment shelves and entered a book-lined office with a view of the park. As he picked up the phone, his businesslike tone of the first few words gave way to a familiar, relaxed patter. Hanging up, he swiveled in his comfortable desk chair and remarked, "That was my broker. He's also my patient. It's the only hold I have over him."

We finished the interview in his office, where he seemed benignly at home, secure enough that he asked my opinion on where medicine should go in the future. When I told him that it still seemed wrong that doctors made so much money, he nodded, understanding. Then he began a more personal explanation of his professional habits, and finally moved to describing his own view of the future.

There are so many obligations which build up in practice, like completing charts, doing rounds, going to committee meetings, and so forth. I concentrate my catch-up on charts to periods when I'm not operating. I finished up forty charts this morning, because I had half an hour between cases. There are another twenty, which I'll find time for when something cancels. But so often, something else comes up—as you know from trying to talk with me three times this week. You just heard the phone ring, and one man is coming over to see me in twenty minutes. The other caller I had to put off until tomorrow. This is a routine kind of thing, even though these aren't my office hours. But you do learn to relax driving in and out in the car, sleeping a little bit because the car knows the way. I catch some sleep at conferences when it is absolutely necessary, and if I am really up against it, I'll take a few days off.

To get where I am now, I became a workaholic. I enjoy my work; it's a pleasure to do all these things, and so I tend not to take many vacations. I'll go to meetings two or three times a year, and take a week off at the time. When my four children are doing something like a play, I'll take time off to go see them, but that's about it.

Almost all of my income derives from my practice. I've found this is about the best investment a doctor can have. I've tried my hand at the stock market, at real estate, and a little bit in banking, but as enthusiastic as I may be, my intelligence is really in the realm of practice, and I'm just like everybody else in the outside world. There are no panaceas for moneymaking—I've lost and gained with every-body else. On the other hand, a lot of investments are tax oriented. With my gross of two or three hundred thousand dollars, and a cost base of a hundred thousand, I am still in the top income-tax bracket, so I'm always looking for a tax oriented investment which would give me some depreciation.

As in every other profession, we surgeons have to keep up with the world. I go to national meetings of surgical associations, and I've also been a delegate to AMA meetings. I think the AMA has the pulse of the American doctor, the practicing doctor—they know his problems. They may not have the pulse of the idealistic young in-tern who isn't aware of what practice is all about, and they may not have the pulse of the full-time fellow and employee of a hospital who is committed to a research and teaching program, but the AMA is made up more of practicing physicians.

As long as we have a capitalist economy, I think there will be a steady, whirling interaction of medicine and society, with ups and downs that will continue, each looking like it is the last moment of the interaction. Ten years from now, things will be much the same, only with more prepaid health plans. There will be more con-straints, more regulations, and the trouble with that is that more medical decisions will be made by panels and committees. Surgery is an art, and the decisions should be made by one person. More people are in the beautiful graveyards because of panel decisions. The panel cannot go in there and examine the patient and make a decision based on true facts; they're making an abstract decision based on a paper construct of what the patient might be, and they're treating the piece of paper.

Socialized medicine would be much worse; it would bankrupt the country. As long as we have a capitalist economy, we're not going to have socialized medicine—even the politicians realize that. The kind of national health insurance which would appeal to the voter is pure pie in the sky. The French have a saying that every time there was a new insurance plan, there was more money for the doctors. This is probably true. Every time a plan is thought up as a political boondoggle to bring in votes—like medicaid and medicare—there have to be enough holes in the plan to let the financially oriented masters of chicanery milk every penny out of it. No plan has ever ended up costing less than it was projected to. Short of a socialist economy, where everybody is on salary, none of the plans is going to save money. They will all just put more money into the system. As long as we stay with capitalism, the doctors will never be truly socialized. As long as you are better and somebody wants you, as in every other aspect of capitalist society, they will pay a little more to get you.

Before the advent of medicare and medicaid, there were top doctors making good incomes, and then there were lots of other doctors who were running around not making very much. My opinion is that while medicare is like private insurance, a reasonable cost system, medicaid is a financial boondoggle—an opiate for the masses and a pile of money for the unscrupulous practitioner. These days most doctors are making more money from the influx of funds from the large plans, and that's why the concept of national health insurance would be a bonanza for the young physician.

On the other hand, the whole country could switch to a socialist economy. It would become like Russia, where the doctors aren't respected, and neither are the executives. The heroes of the Soviet Union are athletes and ballet dancers and top politicians. It's a different ball game. What's happened in Britain is that the best British doctors are right here in New York City, with nice offices. So are the best doctors from Canada. As long as there's a place for them to flee to, they'll go. If I have to, I'll do the same thing. I can speak English, and I can always go to some other country.

If nothing changes that drastically, the other shifts in medicine won't pertain to me. I'm superannuated in the competition. No matter what anybody does, my practice at this point is based primarily on outside doctor and patient referral, and I'm fully booked. I'm not going to get less busy. I'm not dependent on hospital-based referrals, which are the initial source of a physician's money, so that the only way the hospitals could control me would be by limiting my practice. By law they can't even do that—I've practiced twenty-five years in one hospital, and for every year I've been there, they owe me a year of privileges. Even if I am taken off service tomorrow, I can still practice for twenty-five years. And I don't plan to practice much beyond seventy-five, because by that time I'll be deaf, blind, and bored.

The Personal Contact

HANS ROOSEN, GENERAL PRACTITIONER

To balance my inquiry into the profit-oriented side of practice, I decided to talk to a physician on the other end of the spectrum—one who appeared to embody the positive qualities of the "kindly old GP." This is the old-fashioned doctor who spends as much time with each patient as possible, reminding one of television's Marcus Welby in the kind of reassurance he gives to personal patients. I was surprised while talking with Dr. Hans Roosen at the way he so closely resembled the myth. Perhaps it was his office, built into the first floor of a former residential house on a quiet side street. Perhaps it was his accent, his rich Swiss tones conjuring up images of a grandfatherly watchmaker who had turned his craftsmanship and human warmth to the practice of medicine. Or maybe it was the dark leather-bound Latin texts of anatomy and physiology that reposed behind the glass doors of the bookcase.

But most likely it was the gentle yet outgoing way that he greeted me and guided me into his office. It contained the usual tools of a general practice—ophthalmoscopes, examining table, scales, bandages, tongue depressors. Dr. Roosen, white-haired but full of vitality—he was a regular on the local ski patrol—began talking slowly, appraising me with sharp but kind eyes that were steady under his bushy eyebrows. Within minutes, he had warmed to his storytelling. He wanted to share much about what it was like to be a doctor, although he cautioned that it might be harder for young physicians who were just starting out to follow the course he himself had chosen.

He was not content to use mere words to describe his practice. With smooth, sure hands and strong arms, he began demonstrating on me his techniques for reducing a shoulder dislocation. Then, reaching for a fine metal probe, he went through the delicate motions of freeing a clogged tear duct. The calm ease and humor that he maintained throughout these demonstrations testified to his determination to maintain both the personal and the technical skills he had gained during forty years of practice.

First of all, let me tell you that I say what I think. I have in many ways an advantage over younger doctors in general practice, as those of us who are established a long time can operate in certain hospitals under what they call the grandfather clause. That means we are more or less allowed by tradition to do procedures which the younger ones would have to go through elaborate testing and elimination to do. I can do surgery to the extent of my knowledge and training, I can do hysterectomies, I can do radical mastectomies, I can take out appendixes and do general types of surgeries, and I restrict myself not to do resections of the intestines. I could do them, but I feel the rarity of this coming up would make the procedure less definite and safe than if I assist someone else. But I can do fractures to a great extent, particularly since I'm working with mountain rescue and ski patrol for many years, very much exposed to accidents and to fractures. I personally know that I have reduced more dislocated shoulders than any orthopedic physician in the city. Since I do it for practically forty years, it is more likely that I have more experience than the man who is new out of medical school, who in order to take care of a fracture must go into an orthopedic-surgery specialty.

This applies to a lot of things. Let's say a patient has an overflowing of tear ducts. Unless a doctor has been trained in this, he will be unable to help—you've got to have the tools, you've got to have the knowledge and the absence of fear of doing it. No general practitioner will probe a tear duct unless he has been shown in his internship or residency how to do it. [He opened a glassed-in bookcase and took out a venerable-looking anatomy text.] Well, if you take a look [he found the plate depicting tear ducts and pointed to a structure] you have the lacrimal gland, where the tears are produced, and they come out little openings on the surface of the upper eye and flow over the eye, and then they're siphoned off through the tear ducts into the lacrimal sac. And the lacrimal sac goes into the nose, in the inferior nasal meatus, going into the general fluid of the nose. Ah [turning a new page], here you see it better. Here is the gland, here are the eyes, the tear is secreted, they flow over the eye, here they are siphoned off hydraulically and go into the inferior nasal meatus. Now the duct goes up and makes a sharp right angle [pointing on my face with his pencil], goes here, goes in here, and then here. In other words, any probe has to go this way and then it has to be turned around this way, and it has to be brought up this way and pushed down—there. There's a little syringe, a blunt needle with a right angle of gold you can put in the tear ducts and flush them out, and that way you can avoid having inflammation in there, you can free the ducts. And if you hadn't been shown how to do that, you wouldn't attempt to do it. Anyone starting general practice today wouldn't even think of trying that—he would send the patient to an ophthalmologist right away.

I was eight years in the hospitals before I went into practice, and so I had the opportunity to look into different fields. I've worked fifteen years on the health-department board for tuberculosis control, so I have good training in chest diseases and am considered by some as a chest man. Working as I do with the ski patrol they think I am a bone man, and patients whom I operate on consider me as a surgeon. And on Friday I delivered a baby, nine pounds twelve and a half ounces—a huge one, practically walked off the table and almost tied his own cord. And to these people I am the obstetrician or family doctor or whatever. And I take care of the baby—to those people I am the pediatrician. So that is general practice. This is simply what you sum up as experience—doing things hundreds, hundreds of times until you simply know them.

It hasn't been hard to keep up with the changes in medicine over the years. I go to classes in continuing education for physicians, which are often very interesting, though for a while they held them after work on Wednesday evenings, and we would all be asleep in the back rows of the lecture hall, even with the coffee they served. But you know the whole practice of medicine is really relations with patients. I don't think patients have changed that much over the years. They are still most grateful when somebody takes the time with them to listen. You have to give the patient an impression that you're not in a hurry, that you want to hear that patient's story. You don't say, "Well, I have five minutes' time for you, Mrs. So-and-So, and then I've got to go." Or, "Oh, Mrs. So-and-So, excuse me, let me ask you some specific questions, ja, you said that already, please don't tell me again."

If you make this kind of breaking off, you will have a very difficult time, but if you say as the patient comes in, "Hey, you've got a fabulous perfume today, what is it? Oh, really? Well, I sure like it, and by the way, Mrs. So-and-So, do you sometimes step on your lashes? They are so long!"

If you make little remarks like that and appreciate the fact that she is a woman first, no matter how unappealing she is to you, you are a lot better off. Then you can come gradually to the things that bring her here. If a person comes in tense, you don't ask right away about her measles or the chicken pox she had as a child, you ask her, "What brings you here? I see you're pretty tired."

Then she comes out with well, she's this and that, and then you say, "Did you have an argument with your boyfriend?" And maybe she'll start shedding tears.

As soon as a woman in your practice starts crying, she feels better. When you feel a tense person, especially a woman, it is a very important thing if you can make words leading her to cry. Often she is forever grateful, and you say, "You know, I think it's awfully nice that you cry. It shows me that you have enough confidence and relaxation that you can let yourself go."

To give you an example, this is what happened on New Year's night. It was very strange. We were at a party near the ski area. The host was a fabulous ski teacher from Canada, a fantastic skier in deep snow. He has a nice house, built by a local man, with a big bathroom, plush on the floor, and a sunken bathtub, and a big sauna out behind. He had about 100 people at the party—all people who skiied around there. I was there with my wife and two of my daughters.

At about eleven o'clock at night, I looked around and my wife was talking to somebody, the girls were talking with somebody, and I saw a woman sitting on the staircase all by herself. She was about thirty years old, and looking kind of sad. Thirty minutes later I saw her sitting by the fireplace, alone again. I had nothing doing so I came over there and sat down and said to her, "How long have you been divorced?"

"Well," she said, "we aren't divorced yet, we are separated. The children are with my husband and we hope to get together again, but how did you know?"

I said, "well, you look so sad, you could be divorced. Nine out of ten people who look like you are divorced."

Oh, she sat up and talked about her children, about how things were going, how she hadn't wanted to come to the party, how she was talked into it. Now she said she was glad she came, she had been feeling so lonesome. And we talked and talked and talked.

After a while, I walked away, and while I was standing with some guy from Scotland a beautiful blond woman, marvelously built and in very scanty dress, came up to me and asked, "Are you a doctor?"

I said, "Yes, I'm a doctor."

"Are you a butt doctor?"

I said, "What do you mean, am I a quack?"

"No," she said, "are you a butt doctor, somebody who looks with his pipes up butts?"

"Oh, I see." I said, "you mean a proctologist."

"Yeah."

"Well, I use a proctoscope, but no, I'm not a butt doctor."

"What kind of a doctor are you, then?"

I said, "I'm in general practice and surgery."

"You do surgery? Do you do plastic surgery?"

"Oh," I said, "sometimes I may do some plastic surgery, but I'm not a plastic surgeon."

"I'm very interested in plastic surgery," she said.

"Yes," I said, "you had a boob job done."

"How did you know?"

"Well, you alluded to it."

"Look," she said, "it was done beautifully, only two weeks ago. You see, when I was seventeen I had a baby and I was coming out like this" [Dr. Roosen curved both his hands through the air in sizeable arcs.] "And then right afterwards I was flat as pancakes!"

"I understand, but you are so pretty that it doesn't make any difference."

"Well, you've got to see it, he did a marvelous job!" And she dragged me to the bathroom and locked the door. Immediately, she undressed and showed it to me. And the guy had done a fantastic job. [Laugh] He had cut around the outer edge and stuffed the silicone saline plastic bag in there and you could hardly see the scar.

"Oh," I said, "it's excellent."

"You've got to feel it," she said.

"Oh sure." And after I felt them I said, "It's just perfect."

At that moment there was a knock on the door. I said, "You'd better button up again!" So she buttoned up, and we both went to the door.

A woman stood there, and I just walked out past her. I'm convinced that my reputation at that ski area has gone sky high!

Outside, I saw my wife standing and I said, "Anna, come over here. Do you see this girl? She had surgery done on her breast."

"Oh," said the girl, "this is your wife?" I said yes. "Oh, she's got to see it too!" And she took my wife into the bathroom.

Later, on the way home, my wife said to me, "She was a real chippy!"

"Maybe so," I answered, "but that surgeon did a good job."

And just before we left the party, the woman I had talked to first, the lonely woman, came over to me and gave me a hearty kiss on my mouth. My wife looked at me and said, "What's that for?"

And I said, "Well, she was very happy." And then we went home.

So ja, this is the sort of thing that happens in my practice.

I tell you one thing about practice. You've got to have something that keeps you interested in a personal life aside from practice. In my case it's mountainclimbing and skiing and classical music and liking women and children. And not feeling in any way that I am superior to others because I am a doctor. I waxed the floor around here two weeks ago, and I like to stop on the highway when there's an accident to see if I can help the state patrol.

You've got to get off that air that as a physician you are on a higher level. As people look at you, they put you in a higher status anyway, you don't have to ask for it, it's automatic. So you can be yourself, you don't have to try and impress people. The fact that you have a license to practice medicine, that you went through certain studies, is already completely sufficient to set you aside from other people. You are in a respected profession.

I believe that the relationship with patients is totally individualistic and depends on the interchange of words between a doctor and a patient. I want to tell you some secret I don't tell other people. [He dropped his voice slightly.] I don't carry any malpractice insurance. Not at all anymore.

I found out that the amount of encroachment by the lawyers, whom I call the socially accepted mafia of this country, is so enormous that the insurance companies make all their rules for nothing; it's useless. With the money I don't spend on malpractice insurance, I can afford to spend more time with my patients. My opinion is that if you practice carefully, informing the patients of everything you do, keeping in contact with them and informing them that you do everything to the best of your knowledge, then you will avoid lawsuits.

The lawsuits come when you are on a high horse and you don't communicate with people, when you treat them as if they were below your standard or something. I believe that if you act like a human being, you don't get lawsuits.

My opinion is that the personal approach between patient and doctor is the only way that medicine can survive. Any interference by agencies, government, laws, and so on is a downfall of medicine. I believe that if the relationship between the individual physician and the patient is grossly interrupted, it's going to be destroyed. If you have a pain, you don't want to have an agency certifying the pain; you want the person who may help you with that pain having the personal contact with you. This is true for anyone who has had a gallbladder attack or has had a fracture or has had to bear a baby. They don't give a damn about all those rules and regulations; they want their physician to contact them and the nurses to be kind to them. This is the only salvation of medicine, the way I look at it.

Healing the Mind

JOHN STAEHLE, "HOLISTIC" PHYSICIAN

Any survey of the approaches that American physicians bring to medical practice would be incomplete without its taking note of the recent trend toward "holism." If traditional medicine represents such basic aspects of Western civilization as a belief in rationalism and the scientific method to solve human problems, more holistic approaches claim to derive from the Eastern philosophical goals of achieving spiritual unity, an inner peace, in order to overcome difficulty.

Even the words "spiritual unity" seem out of place in a discussion of traditional medicine, and many doctors I spoke with seemed nervous enough about the whole business. "Did you read the editorial in last month's *Journal of the American Medical Association?*" one physician asked me pointedly. "It was titled 'Holistic Medicine— Medicine or Quackery?' Well, that's the question that I ask about it."

Certainly the holistic-health movement has popularized a wide variety of remedies—from massive doses of vitamins to wheat-grass enemas—that seem questionable in value. But in its best form, it represents a willingness to consider forms of therapy—from acupuncture to nutrition—that despite their possible worth have been locked in a closet by a medical profession that moves cautiously toward whatever is not rigidly scientific. At the turn of the century, herbal medicine was part of the repertoire of almost every GP, yet in the push to establish allopathy as the only legitimate medical philosophy (thereby discrediting naturopathy, homeopathy, chiropractic, and a scattered assortment of other schools and cults), herbs were abandoned in favor of more purified, more powerful drugs.

Because I have restricted the interviews in this book to M.D.'s— graduates of allopathic, Flexnerian medical schools—I wanted to find a physician who was sympathetic to the holistic approach but who had remained inside the medical fold. It would have been easy to locate naturopaths, homeopaths, or chiropractors willing to tell me where American medicine had failed. I was more interested in why a medical doctor should choose to go beyond the skills of his training to question them and to define an approach that actively combines the best of traditional and holistic beliefs.

When I met Dr. John Staehle, I knew this search was over.

The Birth Clinic was a one-story structure of dark wood and glass that sat in the shadow of the large suburban hospital. From the out-side, the clinic resembled the sort of professional building that can be found at the edge of a town's business center or shopping mall. Behind the mahogany doors was an equally familiar-looking waiting room with plush chairs, a table with magazines, and a receptionist's station still lined with Christmas cards from patients.

But on the wall above the comfortable chairs was a modern paint-ing of a pregnant woman, with swirls of line and color suggesting her swollen belly, her ovaries, her uterus, and the fetus within. This was the first hint that something about this clinic was different.

Dr. John Staehle greeted me in his office at the end of a carpeted hall. It was late afternoon, but he showed no signs of fatigue. We had met two years before, when the Birth Clinic was only in the planning stages. In a Texas-flatland drawl he had outlined his hopes for a clinic that would allow women to have a choice about what birthing method to use. "The clinic," he had told me in his playful but assured way, "will exist around the conception that birth is a divine event, that we are ushering in a divinity, opening up a place for God to express himself. It will honor the infant as being totally aware and perceptive, a psychic sponge that needs to be handled and treated as such.

"There are many philosophies about how a birth should take

place. LeBoyer recommended a dark room, with a bath of warm water to put the baby in after delivery, and everyone in the room keeping their voices quiet. "Birth without violence,' he called it, and this is the method I would prefer for my personal satisfaction and the child's sake. But if the parents want something else, I am willing to support them in whatever way is appropriate. The clinic will have the services of an obstetrician in town who does a lot of LeBoyer deliveries and has similar ideas about the birth process. We'll have all the medical backup, and if there are any emergencies, Caesarians, whatever, we will be only minutes from the hospital. And we'll use rigid screening criteria to make sure that the women we are working with are healthy, keeping the chances high that their deliveries will be normal. We will hold classes on nutrition, and exercises for natural childbirth. We will teach them relaxation, deep breathing, and how to work with fear, since that is the biggest problem. In most home deliveries, the labor time is much shorter than in a hospital, primarily because in a hospital the mother's fear tightens her muscles. Imagine coming to the hospital to have your first child and being rushed to the delivery room, where it's up in the stirrups, anesthesia, episiotomy, and so on. Of course, if a mother comes to our clinic and it looks like her birth will be high-risk, we'll plan to have it in the hospital delivery room, but still trying for the most natural type of delivery."

Two years later, Dr. Staehle was eager to show me the realities that had come from those dreams. He stood up and walked past me into the hall, moving his large frame with an easy grace. Soft corduroy pants and a red cotton pullover conveyed a further impression of his relaxedness.

We walked past several examining rooms of the standard variety. A poster on one wall said, "No smoking, babies growing." "Someone has to have a lot of strength," said Dr. Staehle, "to go through our childbirth program and still smoke. We really discourage it. We also discourage our mothers from using alcohol, and make sure that they are getting 75 to 100 grams of proteins a day as well as eating lots of unprocessed foods."

The large room at the end of the hall resembled a master bedroom. A wide bed with a patterned quilt stood against the wall, and the air was still and fragrant. Dr. Staehle turned on a bank of overhead fluorescent lights, then flicked them off and instead turned on a smaller set of dim lights. "We try to avoid having births in a brightly lit room," he said. He pushed another button, and a motor whirred, raising the head of the bed. "It's totally mechanical; the mother can be at whichever position is most comfortable."

Near the door was a heat-lamp apparatus on wheels. "It's the same type of baby warmer that's in hospitals," Dr. Staehle said, moving it closer to the bed to show how it could fit over a newborn like an awning. "You take this thermocouple"—he held up an electric button on a cord—"and place it on the baby's skin. The heater's thermostat keeps the baby's environment at a constant temperature. It's fantastic." He bent down and opened the lid of the only other piece of furniture in the room, a cherry-wood antique bureau. The bureau turned out to contain an oxygen tank and other resuscitation tools, syringes, and a typed card of protocol for emergencies. The shiny equipment jarred with the softness of the room's atmosphere until he closed the lid again.

Through the next doorway was a small room where the family could relax during long labors. There was even a refrigerator and sink. The next room was another birthing room like the first, and then there was a comfortable bathroom with a spacious shower. "Usually the mother feels like taking a shower after the birth," Dr. Staehle explained. "The mother stays in the clinic for about four hours after delivery. Then, if there are no complications, she can take her baby home."

We had come to the staff lounge, with another refrigerator and a couch that could be converted to a bed if a doctor or nurse needed sleep during a mother's labor. A chart five feet wide showed the days of the upcoming year and indicated when certain mothers were due to give birth.

"We've got about fifteen births scheduled for January," Dr. Staehle said, sinking into the couch, "and only ten or so in February. Then March is way up, for some reason, with almost thirty births planned. The clinic has been going for almost a year now, and we've had over 100 births. We're working up to an eventual capacity of 30 births a month, which we will share among the three doctors. Bill is the obstetrician I've told you about, and the two other doctors are Jacqueline and myself, both family doctors trained in obstetrics. Each of us will be responsible for 10 or 11 births a month, so we'll only have to work three to four days a week. I'm trying to keep time in my life for the things which are as important to me as medicine. One of those is fathering—have you seen a picture of my son?" He pointed to a snapshot on the wall of a rosy-checked infant breast feeding while a smiling mother looked down at him through blond curls. "My wife, Diana, works here too; she teaches the parenting classes. So, for half the week, I stay at home as the primary parent. And then," he grinned, "I spend a lot of time just playing. It's tempting, though, to spend most of my time at the clinic. Getting it started has been a labor of love for everyone involved."

A bright-eyed nurse in her late twenties leaned in through the doorway to tell Dr. Staehle that a couple had arrived for their first biweekly visit.

In one of the examining rooms, a man and a woman looked up, smiling, as Dr. Staehle walked in. He greeted them and took out the mother's medical chart. "So," he said, speaking in a more serious tone than before, "you've decided to have a natural childbirth, and Dr. Woods saw you last week, and he said you're eighteen weeks pregnant?" The plump young woman nodded.

Dr. Staehle leaned back against the sink and counter beside the door and looked up from the chart. "I don't see anything in your medical history which would give complications, other from the fact that this is your first birth."

The woman giggled.

"Now, you know that we'd like you to gain twenty-five pounds by the end of your term, and it says here that you've signed up for our childbirth-education classes. Do you have any other questions before I take a listen for the baby's heartbeat?"

"Well," she said, "my lower back is starting to hurt me. Can you tell my why?"

"If you're eighteen weeks pregnant, that means that your backbone is starting to go through a lot of changes to get ready for the extra weight it will have to carry. After all, your vertebrae are stacked up like poker chips" (he put one large fist on top of the other to demonstrate). "When they get pulled forward by the added weight of the growing baby, the whole stack of vertebrae, especially the lower ones, begins to bend forward. That can hurt, especially if you don't begin strengthening the muscles of the lower back. Do you know how to rock your pelvis?"

Both husband and wife shook their heads.

"What sort of work do you do?" Dr. Staehle asked her.

"I work in an office all day, just sitting and not getting exercise."

"Most people," Dr. Staehle explained, "keep their pelvis locked in position all the time. But you have to let it become supple." He put his hands on his hips and pushed his own pelvis back and forth. "I know it's not acceptable to do that in public," he said, getting onto his hands and knees on the floor, "but you've got to start loosening and strengthening that joint. Tonight, I want you to do twenty of these." He wiggled his pelvis toward and away from the floor, looking up at the woman without embarrassment. "By the end of the week you should be able to do sixty, and within a month I want you to be doing 120 a day." He got to his feet and took down a stethoscope from the rack on the wall. "Now, we should be able to hear your baby's heartbeat."

The man's head jerked up. "The other doctor listened for it last week," he said with a trace of tightness in his voice, "and he couldn't find it."

Dr. Staehle nodded and picked up an obstetric stethoscope that ended in a short curve of black plastic. The curly-haired woman lay back on the examining table and lifted her shirt to expose her abdomen. Dr. Staehle bent over her and placed the stethoscope on her belly. The room was suddenly quiet as he listened in one location, then moved the stethoscope an inch to the side.

The third spot that he listened to made him smile. "I just got kicked," he said.

"Thank goodness," said the woman.

Minutes later, Dr. Staehle stood beside the nurse at the receptionist's desk, watching the couple walk out the door into the dark winter evening. "I really love them," the nurse said. She had performed the initial history and physical on the woman two weeks ago.

"They're good people," Dr. Staehle agreed.

On a bulletin board was a list of the day's patients. Dr. Staehle had already seen ten patients, mostly mothers in for routine prenatal or postnatal checkups. "This woman was in for a U.R.I. [upper respiratory infection]," he said, pointing to a name, "and this next woman was in with recurrent vaginitis. I talked with her about what was going on in her life, and it turned out she wasn't getting along with her husband. She couldn't tell him how angry he made her. So I showed her how her vaginitis stemmed from her unforgiveness, her unwillingness to let go of those feelings, to put them behind her and allow herself to love him."

Another patient was waiting in an examining room. When Dr. Staehle entered, five-month-old Damien was crawling across the top of the baby scale while his father looked on. Damien was in for a well-baby exam, and his father had brought a list of questions from the mother, who was attending a karate class that night. Staehle listened to the baby's chest with a stethoscope and screwed up his face to make him smile. With a fluid motion, he scooped the baby up and let him waddle along the floor to check for muscle strength and coordination. The father asked some questions concerning how plump Damien was, and Dr. Staehle assured him that everything was within normal limits. He told the father to congratulate the mother for breast feeding so well. The husband asked about switching to a bottle and about beginning to give the baby cow's milk.

"That's fine," said Dr. Staehle, "but keep on eye on Damien as you do so. Cow's milk is one of the most allergenic foods, and many babies develop a rash from it. If that happens, I'd suggest one of the formulas with soya protein. Oh, and by the way, in a month or so Damien should start experiencing stronger anxiety. He'll become a lot shyer, and I just want you to know about it."

"I know," said the father, "we've been reading Brazelton's book on child care." He and Dr. Staehle discussed a few of the other child-care books that the father had heard of, and then Dr. Staehle said good-bye.

"You've got a very healthy baby there," he said.

"He's 'cuting' us half to death," laughed the father.

The last patient was sitting in the waiting room and got up with a start when Dr. Staehle called her name. On the way to his office, she stumbled and apologized. She was in for her first physical examination, and Dr. Staehle had scheduled the last hour of his workday to talk with her.

We took seats in his small, carpeted office. On one wall was the usual bank of physician's diplomas: bachelor of arts, a master of arts, his M.D., his license to practice medicine and surgery, his recognition as diplomate by the National Academy of Family Physicians. These conventional objects were counterbalanced by a curious-looking straw hat hanging on the wall behind Dr. Staehle's chair. It was of a type worn by the natives in Nepal, he told me later: conical in the center of its brown circumference, lifting out from the wall like a deeply tanned breast. It was a small token of the months Dr. Staehle had spent in India and Nepal studying philosophy and religion.

The woman sitting stiffly in her chair began to talk. Pale and dark-haired, she spoke quickly, moving her thin hands. "I'm originally from North Dakota, but I moved to this city six months ago. Now I'm pregnant again, and I'm interested in a natural childbirth."

Dr. Staehle was looking at her chart. "You seem awfully young to have had three children already," he said.

She nodded vigorously. "I'm twenty-four," she said. "My first was when I was seventeen, then one at nineteen, and one at twenty."

Dr. Staehle gazed at her steadily. "All vaginal deliveries, I see from the chart, no complications. And now they live with their father in North Dakota?"

Her speech became more halting. "It was hard to give them up," she began, "but I wasn't making enough money by myself, and I was going to school and I knew he could give them a more stable home life. Still, I wonder about it sometimes. I haven't seen them in a year, and I miss them. And I'm not sure that I totally trust my ex. He's got different ideas about the way children should be raised. You could say he's a religious fanatic."

"I can understand," put in Dr. Staehle, still looking at her carefully, "that's it's hard, but I think you're going to have to say to yourself, 'It's done, I made that decision, and I'm going to live with it.' "

"Oh, I know that, I can accept that," she said, shifting her position slightly; "it's just that the children were a big part of my life."

"I see here also," said Dr. Staehle, "that you were raped last year." His voice was calm. "Would you like to tell me about it?"

"It was something that . . . well, it was a total surprise, for one thing, to be sitting home alone on the couch watching TV, and suddenly someone has come in the back door and is pressing a knife to your throat."

"Did you know him?" Dr. Staehle asked.

"No, and maybe if I'd seen it coming I could have been a little better prepared. I never expected something like that to happen to me, you know? I was so sure that he was going to kill me."

"Did you prosecute?"

"The police never found him." She choked off a bitter laugh. "A clear set of fingerprints off the back door, and they couldn't locate him."

"But you did take it to the police—you didn't try and keep it hidden that this had happened?"

"No, I did everything I could. It happened in North Dakota, but I told the police when I moved that I was willing to come back and testify if they ever caught him. There's been no word. So the only time I keep it inside is with my new husband. He feels guilty that he wasn't there to protect me—he was away on business."

The phone in Dr. Staehle's office was ringing. He answered it and excused himself for a minute. The woman sat in her chair and talked with me about why she wanted a natural childbirth for her fourth child. During her last labor, a resident had refused to give her any pain medication, telling her not to complain so much. She had felt insulted, abused.

Dr. Staehle came back in and sat down, apologizing for the interruption. "I was just about to say when the phone rang that you seem very willing to talk about the rape and about giving your children to your ex-husband. That's good, and before we proceed any farther, I want to ask you if you feel ready to let go of those feelings, to keep them from interfering with this next birth."

"Oh, yes, I think I am. I just wanted to tell you that those were hard experiences for me."

"Okay, fine," Dr. Staehle said, dropping his eyes. "I hope you can talk with me whenever those feelings come up. I want to help you deal with them. Let's have you go to the examining room, and I'll be in in a few minutes to give you your physical."

He stood up, showed the woman to another room, and handed her a white examining smock. While she undressed, we returned to Dr. Staehle's office. I asked him how often it was necessary to turn away a prospective mother.

"Almost never," he replied. "The only two criteria we use are willingness to attempt a natural childbirth of some kind, and ability to pay our fee of 1,000 dollars. We take mothers at all levels of pregnancy risk. If they are at high risk, we'll have the birth in the hospital rather than trying to have her deliver here."

I asked Dr. Staehle if the clinic took patients on welfare.

"Generally not," he said. "For one thing, medicaid currently pays the physician only 50 percent of usual and customary fees. My overhead alone is more than that, so I would lose money if I saw welfare patients. The only way I could afford to see them would be if I whipped them in and out in fifteen minutes, and I'm not willing to practice like that. I've got some other, more philosophical objections to treating welfare patients, but we can talk about that later."

We went back to the examining room and Dr. Staehle knocked on the door. When we entered the patient was sitting on the examining table, wearing her white smock and a nervous expression.

Dr. Staehle walked up to her and took her chin in his hands. "I'm going to run through a normal screening physical," he explained, working his hands along her jaw and neck. "I'm also going to order some blood tests, since you seem a little anemic. Your face and conjuctiva are a bit pale."

"I've always been pale," she said.

"Have you enrolled in a birthing class yet?" he asked, lifting up her hair to look in her ears with an otoscope.

"Yes, but I wanted to ask you about nutrition. My husband wants you to give me a strict diet to follow. He says I eat too much junk food."

"I'm not going to do that," he said, helping her lie back and palpating her breasts for lumps. "I'll give you a copy of our list showing what foods contain which nutrients, and then you and he can work out the best diet. By the way, I don't think you'll have any problem breast feeding. Your breasts are healthy and the glands are good-sized. Now, I'm going to examine your cervix and do a Pap smear."

The woman groaned and lay back, putting her feet on the cushioned supports. Dr. Staehle reached into the supplies cupboard for a speculum and ran the shiny metal tool under warm water in the sink before turning back toward the woman. Explaining each procedure to her, Dr. Staehle inserted the speculum and brought his examining light closer. "I can see your cervix now," he said. "Have you ever seen it before?"

"No."

He reached back into the cupboard and took out a hand mirror with a sky blue handle. He placed it in the woman's hand and showed her how to hold it.

"You should be able to see the opening of the cervix," he said, adjusting the light for her. She was turning the mirror from side to side, a look of fascination on her face. "You have what's called a fish-mouth cervix. Instead of there being a tiny opening, yours makes an upside-down U because it's expanded each time you had a baby. Now I'm going to do a Pap smear." He took a small wooden stick and inserted it into her cervical opening through the speculum, rotated it once, then removed it, smeared mucous on a slide, and placed the slide in a small plastic jar. With an equally smooth and rapid motion, he swabbed her cervix with a cotton swab to test for venereal disease. Then he removed the speculum and gently felt for her uterus by inserting two fingers in her vagina and pressing on her abdomen with his ungloved hand. "You're pregnant, all right," he said. And then the exam was over. "Before you leave," he said, "have the nurse test a little of your blood for anemia. Good night, now."

It was eight o'clock in the evening, but Dr. Staehle still seemed fresh. We walked back to his office and sat down. I asked him how he had chosen to be a physician, and how he had come to be different from the norm.

As Dr. Staehle talked, he began to spin out ideas that left the realm of the practical and rational. He spoke more slowly, searching for the correct words.

I went to college in Houston to become a Baptist minister, but basically didn't find anyone that I saw eye to eye with. I was a freshman in college, the whole world was wide open to me for study, and I began to question everything. Just questioning, questioning, questioning, questioning; I don't believe this; I don't believe that; I believe this; I don't believe that; and I didn't have anybody who thought that was okay. The people going into the ministry were a different breed; they were all alike, and I was different, so I figured something was wrong with me. I got more and more disenchanted and angry and thought the church was really missing it. I extended this to all religion, threw out the baby with the bath water, and became totally bitter.

I became a Marxist and ended up getting a master's degree in sociology. Then I found a community, a place in which I went and spewed out all of my negativity and anger. They said, "Far out, that's great and we love you." So, within a loving, supportive community I was able to experience the warmth of human beings exploring together, and I didn't have to have a particular belief, so then I started looking at what of the baby that I had thrown out did I want to take back. That was a long process, over years, but my religion began to be universal, I looked at other religions, other philosophies.

I was still interested in people, so I entered pre-med at that time—started taking biology and chemistry. Then, when I went to medical school, I was impressed with how much social factors impinged on biological and medical matters, so I headed towards psychiatry. That was the time that family practice was making a comeback, and that really met my needs as a specialty, because the emphasis was on the whole person, on the patient's social milieu.

As a family practitioner, I do a lot of what a minister does. Most of the people who come in are what is known as the "worried well." Probably the largest disease that people suffer from is spiritual deprivation. This is characterized by the people who have everything they could possibly want—they have "made it" by any traditional standards, and yet they have a sense of anomie; they're not satisfied or happy.

There are different ways to work with them about this, teaching them to let go of their problems, get off it, to see that the choice they are making is not bringing them health and happiness. Most of my patients respond well to my approach, but I don't necessarily spill the whole bag of beans to everyone who walks into the office. There are different levels that people are willing to hear. They come in for a Band-Aid, and they might not want to hear my conception of how the universe is glued together. So I give them a Band-Aid. And other people are truly spiritually deprived, and when I spring that on them and suggest that perhaps that is what's going on, often they are just delighted.

A lot of times their story just comes out, and by telling it to another person, the meaning becomes obvious to them: they'll put two and two together. For example, they will see how their migraine headaches are created by their father drinking. The first time he started drinking they didn't think about it, and the second time they didn't realize that was the time they started having migraine headaches. But they put their story out, and you start asking them questions, and they see that essentially what they're got is a problem of nonforgiveness. They are holding on to their anger and resentment toward their father, and they are not forgiving him, turning him loose, letting him be, until by a process of forgiveness they can be turned loose of the pain and the problems they are holding on to in their head.

I teach people how to meditate, to love themselves twenty-four hours a day whether they want to or not. I urge people to get a good amount of exercise every day, and I work with them on their diets, on nutrition, getting them feeling well, feeling good.

I haven't been around long enough to know if people get dependent on me. I'm real active trying to get people dependent on themselves, because I think it's essential they recognize that their mind is their own physician, that true healing comes from within.

This makes them angry sometimes, and that is a subtle dance, because it doesn't serve me or them for them to be getting angry over what I'm saying. That is the art of medicine—to convey information so that the other person can hear it and not get defensive. Occasionally I will still be a little brash, say something a little too quick, or point out something that they are not ready to hear, and then if they become defensive, well, it's all over for that encounter. Thay will have to wait for some other time to hear it. And if they never hear it, they get to live out their life as a victim, and if they're miserable and don't have a good time, that's real sad.

The reason I don't like working with welfare patients is that even before they come to me, they've put themselves into a victim role. They are letting society say to them, "Yes, you can't help yourself; yes, you need public assistance." If they can't help themselves financially, if they see themselves as helpless, how are they going to be able to work on getting well? My experience is that they aren't willing to work with me on this. They expect me to cure them.

These people are turning and turning around, caught in circles, staying below the surface of emotional and physical wellness. But now and then [Dr. Staehle contorted his body and stretched out his arm] they get a hand out from the muddle and wave it around a bit. If they're lucky, they'll be able to grab a hand and help themselves up. I can see myself helping with that role. I don't believe there is anyone who can't help himself, who is a true loser. But if someone isn't willing to question their victim role, they won't be able to take advantage of what I have to offer.

I'm certainly not going to feel guilty about those people. I think that guilt is one of mankind's most worthless emotions. And I saw during my training that American medicine puts people, especially poor people, into helpless positions and tries to keep them there. If things are going to change, those people have to become less dependent, and that's not going to happen if the government keeps pouring money into welfare and medicaid.

You see, my philosophy has changed from the days when I was a Marxist. Marx believed that if you change the system, individuals would take more control of their own lives. But I'm sure now that you can't bring in social responsibility and hope that people will later learn some personal responsibility. Marx thought that the proletariat were all revolutionaries at heart. Well, that turned out to be untrue.

So, I don't support the medicaid system. It's just a choice I had to make somewhere along the line.

I think that the only thing medicine can accomplish is the healing of the patient's mind, and whatever can be given to a person to facilitate that healing should be used. That can mean antibiotics, or anti-inflammatory medication, any number of those pharmaceuticals that we use in the medical profession, since what we are really doing is healing the mind. We work with both parameters, the external and the physical environment, and how we as whole persons interact with our environment. It is true that penicillin is specific against certain microbes, and it makes sense to use an appropriate antibiotic, but if a person at some point within that play in which they are taking the antibiotics doesn't conceive himself as well, then he is just leaving himself open again. I mean, how did the bacteria get in? The bacteria is invited in. When I have a cold, it means that I have invited a cold virus in. Now, I don't know how I did that, but it helps me to look at things. Usually I can come up with some decision that I made, since at every point of sickness there is a decision made to be sick. The trick is that we are naturally well, naturally whole—that's the state in which our universe was created—and at some point we tend to separate ourselves from that perception of wholeness.

I was trained to be a body technician, to look at the body, to test it in all its humors, and to come up with some diagnosis, and to treat it at that level. Most medical treatment is at the symptoms level:

replace that, kill this, kill that, make it well, wipe it out. And then that's it—they get people from being critically ill to being asymptomatic, but there is a whole range above that, increasing levels of wellness leading up to what Abraham Maslow talked about with "self-actualization," and then to what I consider to be the highest point, which is God-realization. This doesn't fit into the thinking of most physicians, but my belief is that we are all basically whole, and within each of us is the memory of that wholeness, of our connection to infinite being. By our egos and our personalities, we separate ourselves from a willingness to hear that truth. In other words, the truth lies within us, is recognizable, and can be heard. But we have negative thought mass that overlies our willingness to do all of that.

I haven't found myself becoming callous because of my work as a physician. In medical school there was the phenomenon of tiredness, and I probably lost my sensitivity for periods of time, feeling the effects of schedule and whatnot. There were times when I wouldn't stand up for my own limits, would work thirty hours and get totally wiped out, and think that I had to. In retrospect, I see that I didn't have to, that I can get out of it if I am willing to stand up for what I know and believe to be true. And I think doctors are a wonderful group of people; we really are just folk [laugh]. We are on the forefront of a lot of issues that have to do with the frailty of the human body, a lot of weighty decisions, and a lot of high expectations from society. All of this goes together to make it a profession where one doesn't have a lot of defenses, so doctors tend to retreat into technological bullshit, which is what most of medicine consists of nowadays.

If you look at it statistically, we really are not prolonging life. I doubt we are even having much effect on morbidity. When you examine a simpler society and see how it functions, there seem to be lots of advantages to letting go of certain things that we currently make a big deal of. I personally believe that it's all right if people die, but each year the country spends millions of dollars on specialized equipment to keep a few people alive who really should be allowed to die.

What my approach to practice really boils down to is life-styling.

If you have a patient come in for a routine visit and you give them an X ray and a physical exam, you haven't done much for them. The method is not cost effective. But if you talk about nutrition and stress levels, and teach them how to take care of themselves, I call it life-styling, and I think it's very effective. It means putting people in the driver's seat with regard to their lives.

The renewed interest in family practice over the last decade is a move toward a holistic approach. A lot of people think that holistic medicine has to be something radically different, that it must involve things like the use of herbal remedies rather than pharmaceuticals. These people say things like "It's okay to use acupuncture, but aspirin is not holistic." Well, I don't agree with them. Just because you use something that is nontraditional doesn't mean that it's more holistic than anything else; the concept has to be broader than that. If you put your faith in herbal teas, that's just as illusory as believing that it's the penicillin that makes you well. I use a lot of standard medical techniques, and while I may feel that acupuncture has a definite role in energy balancing, I also think Western medicine has its contribution. We have to open ourselves to using all the methods, at the same time realizing that what we are dealing with is delusion.

The nurse knocked on the door to tell Dr. Staehle that the new patient's blood hematocrit showed mild anemia. After he thanked her, I asked Dr. Staehle how he felt about a recent AMA resolution stating that all births should take place only in hospitals under the guidelines of the American Obstetrics and Pediatrics Associations, in the interest of reducing risk.

"It's going to be a while," he said, "before the rest of the medical community accepts these new ideas. Doctors are a cautious group, and in a way that's how it should be. The local physicians were cool to us at first, but recently they've started to see how successful our approach is, and how committed we are to making it work. If I was back in Texas, the local medical society would probably have tried to kick us out by now. But this city is filled with more progressive, thinking human beings.

"And I'm used to being different in the way I practice medicine. When I was a freshman in medical school, they put us through a battery of psychological testing. When the results came back, they recommended that I see a psychiatrist, that there was something very wrong with my attitudes. But you know, the Gaussian curve has two extremes [Dr. Staehle traced a bell-shaped curve on the wall]. Both are deviations from the norm. Now on one extreme, you've got a few real crazies and idiots, and on the other, there are an equally small number of gifted people. It's sometimes hard to distinguish the two [laugh], but I think when enough time has gone by that we'll be seen as being in the gifted category."

PART IV

Researchers

"Medicine is part and parcel of modern science. The human body belongs to the animal world. It is put together of tissues and organs, in their structure, origin, and development not essentially unlike what the biologist is otherwise familiar with: it grows, reproduces itself, decays, according to general laws. It is liable to attack by hostile physical and biological agencies; now struck with a weapon, again ravaged by parasites. The normal course of bodily activity is a matter of observation and experience; the best methods of combating interference must be learned in much the same way. Gratuitous speculation is at every stage foreign to the scientific attitude of mind."

—Abraham Flexner, *Medical Education*

When Flexner advocated that doctors possess above all the qualities of the scientist, he was acting in the same deterministic scientific faith that has inspired rationalist philosophers since the Englightenment: that scientific knowledge, properly applied to human problems, could usher in a new age of civilization.

This optimism has a strong basis in medicine. The germ theory of disease made possible the progress in immunization and antibiotics that had such a dramatic effect on epidemic diseases in the early twentieth century. Yet this was only the beginning.

Germ, antibiotic, immunization—the agent, the cure, the prevention. These are the guidelines along which medical research functions. Isolate the causative agent for a disease, thereby determining the "etiology." Study that agent—virus, bacterium, antigen, poison, whatever. Through an understanding of the agent's strategy against the human organism, correct that damage with some form of antidote. Better yet, stop the sore throat, the diarrhea, the cancer, before it has even begun by preventing the agent from gaining access to vulnerable bodies.

This is logic at work, trying to make sense out of the complicated affair of human illness. At its best it is pure, cold, inductive. But it doesn't always lead easily to the answer. There is a long list of diseases bearing the uncomfortable label "idiopathic"—of unknown etiology. And what then?

The three researchers who tell their stories, who describe their approaches to research, represent the different crossing points of cure and prevention, discovery and perplexity. One describes how it felt to be part of the postwar research boom in the development of cures, and where he feels that boom has led. Another has concentrated on prevention, by looking specifically at the role of stress in producing disease and how it can be controlled. The final researcher demonstrates how he has waged a personal war with the unknown by refining his technique of organ transplantation to a repeatable, reliable science, despite his admission that he does not yet know why his technique works. His empirical perfectionism is his personal way of dealing with the inadequacy of present knowledge in his field, one that he feels will in time lead to new discoveries.

Medical research has ushered in a dazzling array of wonder drugs, miracle surgeries, and innumerable medical facts. Yet each new discovery can raise new questions: what exactly *is* a virus? *Why* do people get one disease and not another? The questions form easily, one after another, sometimes overshadowing the answer that sparked them. A noted researcher stood on a porch during a cocktail party, gazing up at the summer stars.

"When I began researching," he mused, "I felt we were on the verge of big breakthroughs into what made people tick. But soon I found myself following more and more closely in the footsteps of previous workers. It was as if a huge problem was lurking out there, and to hide from it I had to move farther into academic examination of smaller, more solvable problems. All because the real mystery," he spread his arms out over his head, as if to hold up some massive weight, "is so limitless as to become terrifying."

Everything in Life
Is Simple

Robert H. Williams, Endocrinologist

Dr. Robert Williams stood with a knot of eager first- and second-year medical students, sharing cider and doughnuts before the start of his morning lecture in endocrinology.

Endocrinology is the study of hormones; those messenger chemicals which exert overwhelming influences over the biological function of higher organisms totally out of proportion to the tiny concentrations in which they occur. To pursue their secrets is to deal daily with the unseen, the underlying. And yet Dr. Williams, one of the most prominent endocrinologists in the world, was a burning fuse of openness and bravado, optimism and expansiveness.

"I want to remind all of you," he was telling the students, "that research is something you can do every day of your lives, whether you go into family practice or get an academic position. Research is only a way to think. So, become researchers, and do your research well, but above all have fun while you're doing it."

He took a sip of cider, then broke into a toothy grin. Despite his graying hair and long white lab coat, his grin might have been that of a young southern boy out squirrel hunting for the first time, full of mischievousness and undaunted curiosity.

"I'm fascinated by every phase of medicine," he announced, "but when I was a boy growing up in Tennessee, my mother wanted me to be a preacher for a long while. My dad wanted me to be a businessman, but since the age of five, I was determined to study medicine. My son told me the other day, 'Dad, you preach to us all the time, and nobody has won a nickel off of you in your life!' So I suppose I made out all right."

From the time I first met him to the last time we talked, those four personae of Robert Williams—the distinguished professor, the boyish explorer, the southern preacher, and the unstoppable businessman—often took turns revealing themselves before finally mingling into one unified, winning personality. It was a personality perfectly suited to the demands of his forty-year career in academic medicine. He had made one breakthrough after another in the understanding of the diseases of the thyroid gland and later in the causes and treatment of diabetes, publishing over 300 scientific articles and finding time to assemble *Endocrinology*, a work that has gained worldwide recognition as the definitive text in the field. In 1947 he left the faculty at Harvard to head the department of medicine at the newly created University of Washington Medical School. To the surprise of medicine departments around the country, he soon turned his department into a national center for medical research and teaching. As one of the luminaries of postwar medical research, he devoted his missionary zeal and persuasive salesmanship to the task of turning the federal resources that had fought Fascism into tools for fighting a peacetime war against disease. In 1954, he could proclaim:

> Never before has clinical research received such a glorified position or as much financial support as today. The public demands it, Congress has provided for it, medical schools clamor for it, and patients not only tolerate it but sometimes request it. Federal support for medical research has climbed from an annual rate of about 18 million dollars in 1941 to 181 million in 1951. This increase is out of proportion to both the increase in trained medical research manpower and the increase in national income. It should be viewed not as today's excess, but as yesterday's deficiency.

Twenty-five years later, Dr. Williams listened to a final question from a student, bending his six-foot frame and adjusting his hearing aid. He had slowed his pace considerably in the last few years, and teaching this class of medical students was one of the joys that his more relaxed schedule afforded him. In addition, he was the director of the university's Diabetes Research Center and was spending a large part of his time doing direct laboratory research on a newly defined digestive hormone called GIP (gastric inhibitory peptide).

The last students took their seats in the large, banked lecture hall. Dr. Williams adjusted the microphone hanging from a cord around his neck. "All right, now, ladies and gentlemen." The southern drawl was full of effort, but each word emerged clear at last. "I want you to meet Linda Farrel, one of my favorite patients. She will fit right into this morning's lecture on the diseases of thyroid gland."

A middle-aged, fleshy woman dressed conservatively in dark blue walked out from the patients' waiting room. Dr. Williams swung his gaze in her direction.

"Linda, I want you to take a seat right here." He extended his arms and guided her into a chair facing the class. Circling behind her, he slowly wrapped his long, steady fingers around her neck, letting his middle fingers touch under her chin. Linda Farrel dropped her eyes to see, then, finding she couldn't, gazed out at the class with a half-smile.

"I want you all to watch closely," Dr. Williams instructed the class, "because no matter what they teach you in your physical-examination class, this is the way to find the thyroid. I've felt many, many thousands of them, and this is how I do it. You locate the laryngeal prominence of the thyroid cartilage—that's easy because it's the Adam's apple—and then move a little lower until you strike the cricoid cartilage. Now, then, go a little ways to the side"—his fingers retreated slightly as he spoke—"and ask the patient to swallow."

Linda Farrel pumped her throat visibly, her features tight.

"And there," Dr. Williams called out, "I can feel her thyroid gland coming up to touch my fingers. What I'm feeling is thyroid cancer."

He paused, looking around the room, which had grown quiet. The students leaned forward for a better look, as if by straining they could stand where Dr. Williams was standing, feel what his fingers could feel.

"Linda has had primary thyroid cancer for some time—I diag-nosed it in her seven years ago. But you're not worried about it, are you, Linda?" He gazed down at her scalp, hands still resting on her neck.

Linda Farrel rolled her eyes, mouthing to the class, "Yes, I am!" There was laughter, and she kept her smile.

Dr. Williams caught her signal. "No, she's not," he said firmly. "Linda, why don't you tell the class what it's been like to have can-cer."

The female voice faltered, then found itself. "It's been very scary, but it's been wonderful having Dr. Williams take care of me. He doesn't let his patients feel sorry for themselves. He tells me to get on with life."

"That's right," Dr. Williams put in, "there's too much living to do. And besides, I've always said that death wasn't so bad. To block out all the pain of death, the brain releases certain hormones, enke-phalins, which are the same hormones released by the hallucin-ogenic drugs. I've been halfway through the pearly gates many times myself, and I can tell you it's an experience full of pretty col-ors, nice smells, warm feelings."

The class was laughing again. Dr. Williams had made his point— death was something to laugh at. Anything that detracted from the fullness of life became the real enemy. Dr. Williams's own en-counters with dying had come in the early 1960s, when he was chairman of the department of medicine and working seventy-and eighty-hour weeks. A blocked coronary artery triggered a series of more than twenty cardiac arrests. The faculty and house staff from the department of medicine stayed by his bedside around the clock, three doctors at a time, interns and tenured professors, ready to apply heart massage and defibrillation. After several days, one of the first temporary Pacemakers ever used in that part of the country was threaded through a vein to his heart, and soon afterward, the heart had repaired itself. Telling me about it later, Dr. Williams could just as well have been describing an enjoyable cocktail party at his lab.

"For a few days, my heart attack was just routine, and then it began to stop, for ten, twenty, twenty-five seconds. Each time that happened, I was dead, for all practical purposes. When the brain is without oxygen like that, you get convulsions, and in fact some of my convulsions were so strong that I got a hernia.

"But between attacks, when my heart had come back, I was immediately conscious. I was either dead or wonderfully alive—there was no pain. My friends were the ones suffering. You see, I had adjusted my philosophy, and I was laughing in between attacks, kidding the fellows taking care of me. Sixty doctors, the whole department of medicine, three of them at a time doing nothing but watching the heart monitor. I could always tell when an attack was coming on. I could sense an aura, and then I'd yell out, 'Boys, it's time to pound my chest again!'

"I've got doctor friends who've had tremendous depressions after a heart attack. They become scared to do anything, but I was walking a quarter of a mile a day within five weeks of my coronary, and within two months I was walking four miles a day."

Dr. Williams and I were talking in his large office, which was half-filled by his huge, battleship gray desk, covered with piles of reprints and textbooks. As we talked, the many phone calls lighting up an intercom console were diverted to his secretary, who nevertheless knocked on the door now and then throughout the several hours of conversation with messages that simply couldn't wait. It was not possible for Dr. Williams to exist for long outside the center of activity. And as he talked, he seemed to actually become that hub of energy and accomplishment. One wall of the office consisted of bookshelves, another was taken up by a picture window, but the other two were studded with enough plaques and certificates to remind one of a Victorian trophy room. The Distinguished Leadership Award from the Endocrine Society, the Outstanding Achievement Award from *Modern Medicine*, an "RH positive" award from his students and co-workers. In between the gold and silver were photographs of researchers who had originally worked under his guidance before going on to head up other departments of medicine, to become deans of medical schools and universities, to make significant discoveries on their own.

Dr. Williams pointed out a few of them, and then because I had asked him to talk about medical research, he explained, "I had only been a research fellow for two months myself when I was offered a full-time faculty position at Harvard, based on the fact that I had published fifteen clinical papers as a house officer. Now, the point is that from the time I assumed that faculty job up until two years ago, I was doing very little of the actual research myself in terms of having the number-one leadership and rolling up my sleeves and working with the test tubes and the chromatography. But I've always had excellent research fellows, and while I was always making suggestions and offering guidance, the quality of my research accomplishments has been very much related to the quality of my research fellows.

"So I had always felt that there was a gap in my career, and so during these last two years, I've done virtually 100 percent of my own research. Oh, I've had technical help, but I've been right in there passing stomach tubes on the dogs that I was working on, doing the intravenous catheterization. Even though I may take on more research fellows in the future, I have a mixed reaction to that now, because when you're the main person doing the work, you don't have to fiddle with anybody else—you go and do the work and then you're done with it. And I get a fascination out of it, and the mere fact that I've been head of the department of medicine and have gotten all sorts of honors hasn't hampered me a bit in running down the corridors with test tubes or cutting rats' heads off or in working with sick people with brain death, where I took every specimen myself, making the incisions when the heart was still beating, and so forth."

He paused, smiling, and sensing the need to provide me with some more background. He talked easily about himself, somehow exuberant without being boastful, as if the wild successes he had enjoyed were commonplace, part of everyone's birthright.

"You see," he explained, "Medicine was just a natural for me, like music is for somebody else. I did quite well in biology and chemistry in college but graduated with only a B-plus average, because I did mediocrely in my other courses—literature, *Beowulf*, all of that—I couldn't care less about them. I had already decided to go to medical school, and so in my senior year I applied to the University of Pennsylvania, my first choice, and Vanderbilt.

Well, July 1, 1929, was a very important day in my life. Although I had already been accepted at Vanderbilt, that day I got a letter from the dean of the University of Pennsylvania medical school saying "Sorry, we can't take you."

"Well," I said to myself, "I'll show them!" I started really turning on the steam. I went to Vanderbilt, got all A's my first year, then transferred to Johns Hopkins and ended up at the top of my class. It was evident to me as soon as I hit medical school that I was right where I belonged.

I had fourteen years of training after high school and really meant to have more. One summer I worked as a traveling salesman to earn money, and got to talk to some doctors out in practice. Almost all of them said to me that if not for their wife and kids they would have stayed in academic medicine. There was so much more I wanted to know, so after my residency I got a fellowship in endocrinology.

I'd only been a fellow for two and a half months, as I said, when I went to a CPC [clinical pathological correlation—a medical conference where autopsy findings are compared with the patient's records] at the Boston City Hospital. They held some of the best CPC's in the country, with great doctors attending. That day I was the only one that hit either of the two diagnosis. One was a gonococcal endocarditis; the other was cancer of the head of the pancreas.

Well, the following week, I got three offers for teaching full-time medicine—from Harvard, Vanderbilt, and Boston University. I went ahead and accepted the job at Harvard. This meant heading up endocrinology at Boston City Hospital, and during my eight years there, I personally cared for 440 thyrotoxics [patients suffering from thyrotoxicosis, an endocrine disorder]. My main goal was to see if I couldn't manage them with a brand-new thiouracil drug. I was the second person in the world to use it, and in doing so, to avoid surgery. This and other research that I coordinated on the thyroid led to less than 10 percent of the patients who would have previously required surgery being operated on for this disorder.

But after twelve years of thyroid research I decided that diabetes was more of a challenge, so soon after I left Harvard and came out here to start the department of medicine, I switched to diabetes as a research topic. The thyroid was just too simple!

At that time, very little was known about insulin [the hormone lacking in diabetes] secretion, distribution, and degradation. My group started out researching all three of those topics. We were the first—Dr. Elgee and Dr. Hogness were working with me then—to show the human distribution of insulin in tissues, and later on to identify the specific enzymes and organs taking part in the degradation process. We found that the liver and kidneys did most of the degradation, through enzymes like insulin transhydrogenase, and this was why patients in kidney failure didn't need as much insulin—their kidneys weren't breaking it down.

The problem of insulin secretion is the most interesting part of all. We showed that obese people secreted more insulin in response to an injection of glucose, even if they were diabetic, than the normal-weight nondiabetics did! So, something was special between obesity and insulin secretion.

About the same time, we were conducting extensive trials of some of the drugs for diabetes—tolbutamide, sulfanilamide, acetohexamide . . . I'd say we published twenty papers on the subject. However, we were also among the first to completely quit using all of these oral drugs, because considering all the good and the bad they do and the great unknown there's just not enough justification to use them.

There was so much research going on around the world that I convinced NIH, though it didn't take much selling, to set up grants for diabetes centers. In order to do the best job in clinical research, you need to have the most appropriate facilities. This means not only excellent hospital resources and laboratories and researchers, but also a diabetes registry where patients are very carefully grouped and you can keep track of some of the rare ones, like lipotrophic diabetes and identical twins with diabetes, very young ones, very old ones, and so on. The British are way ahead of us on the registry idea—they've been doing it for years.

Starting about three years ago I got a group of eight specialists together: virologists, immunologists, pathologists, geneticists, diabetologists, and others, in order to work with juvenile-onset diabetes [one of the two major forms of diabetes], starting as soon as a child is diagnosed and then doing extensive studies to evaluate their medical and genetic background. Eventually we hope to pick out the ones who might get juvenile-onset diabetes before they get it. You see, there is evidence to suggest that this form of diabetes might result from an infection, especially with the Coxsackie virus. We've been culturing patients for Coxsackie virus and measuring antibody titers against the Coxsackie virus, and in fact we've found that many juvenile-onset diabetics have an antibody deficiency against Coxsackie virus, so that while both diabetics and nondiabetics commonly get infected with Coxsackie virus, those with an immune deficiency will tend to get diabetes. And this is the kind of a study you can only do if you have a large number of patients to work with.

Right now we're on the verge of a great resurgence in clinical research with the adult-onset diabetic [the other predominant form]. The preliminary research has been going on for several years. It ties back to what I said about obesity and insulin secretion. The insulin is produced by cells in the pancreas called Beta cells. Expert pathologists have found that adult-onset diabetics have at least 50 percent of the normal number of Beta cells. We know from our surgical colleagues that you have to remove more than 85 percent of Beta cells from a normal person to produce diabetes, so the problem is not in the Beta cells, as was previously thought.

A lecture that was given last month at the International Diabetes Federation by Dr. Pike talked about Claude Bernard's observation 100 years ago that if you injure a mammal's brainstem, you can cause diabetes within several hours, so there is some tie between higher brain centers and insulin secretion. I'm in the middle of investigating this. I just finished a chapter for the sixth edition of my textbook *Endocrinology*—the most difficult chapter I've ever written. It concerns the interrelationship of gastrointestinal hormones [one of the hormones released by the intestinal tract during digestion of food] with the brain and the pancreas. Almost all of these gastrointestinal hormones on this list here have been shown to also increase insulin output. [He handed me a slip of paper which had been taped to the wall above the desk, as if in preparation for the interview. On it was written in a bold hand:

Cholecystikinin
Secretin
Neurotensin
Substance "P"
Vaso-inhibitory Peptide
Motilin
Gastrin
Acetylcholine]

Well, almost every one of these hormones is also found in the brain. We think they are affecting appetite centers. We were the first to show that Beta endorphins increase the appetite, whereas Bombassin definitely inhibits appetite. So I'm continuing to investigate this, and also collaborating with the psychologists on the study of these hormones, especially the catecholamines and the gastrointestinal hormones, as they affect food intake. Virtually all adult-onset diabetics are obese, and they stay obese no matter what you say to them. And take the fact that almost 50 percent of the Pima Indians in Arizona have diabetes. If you go back in their history one hundred years, you'll find very little incidence of diabetes. But the white settlers cut off the drainage of a river and changed the whole life pattern of the Indians. Now most of them are fat. I visited down there and the doctor showing me around told me, "Bob, when you walk around today, no matter what time of day it is you'll see all the Indians eating!" And he was right. It's just like the desert rat—this animal has no diabetes when he lives in the desert, but if you bring him into the laboratory and feed him rich food, he will get diabetes.

So the eating response is tied up here [he tapped his head], and somehow the hormones in the gut affect it. So we're looking vigorously for a compound that will inhibit the appetite center so that people with diabetes will lose their desire for food.

In the next few years, I plan to deeply involve myself in psychoendocrinology—the study of how hormones affect the brain. There's no question about how behavior is determined by the chemical balance of the body. If I blocked your RNA and protein synthesis, which I can easily do with certain drugs, you could come in here today and tomorrow you couldn't tell me one word I told you, because all your memory depends on the synthesis of those chemicals. Lots of hormones affect memory and recall; steroids, thyroid homone, to say nothing of the neurotransmitters like acetylcholine. And there's a lot of evidence to indicate that if you alter a person's metabolism of serotonin and enkephalins, you can cause all sorts of schizophrenic reactions and mental depression. If this is true, just how far are you going to get by having a schizophrenic person lie on a couch and talk about himself?

As a medical student, my professor of psychiatry was Adolf Meyer, one of the greatest psychiatrists this country has ever had. One of the questions he asked us was this: If you pick up a cat on a street, take him to the laboratory, and somehow reproduce that cat in your laboratory, atom for atom, molecule for molecule, when you are finished would that reproduced cat be alive, and would he have the same thoughts as the cat you picked up on the street? Well there's no question on earth about it!

In the next few years, I want to begin studying prisoners, lining up collaborators in psychology to do psychometric testing, and so forth. I have a very different attitude from most of the public toward criminals. My feeling is that some of them are so *sick* and so beyond cure in the light of present information that instead of saying, "You mean SOB, you killed fourteen people, now you will hang until your last breath," my reaction is "I feel very sorry for you, you're a very sick person. To avoid so much suffering on your part through being confined for years to come, my recommendation, though I won't force it on you, is to offer you the opportunity of any form of termination. It could be a large dose of nembutal, or gas. You'll die with less suffering than most people who die a natural death." I'd say that, because I don't think that death is the worst punishment. I think that life imprisonment is far worse, and that through it so many people are far more agonized than if they had the chance for termination, particularly if someone conveyed it to them, that death would be a very easy deal. Now of course this would only be for the criminals who are apparently incurable.

I developed my philosophy of death and dying long ago, even before I had my coronaries. I practiced euthanasia on my dad in 1941. For years I had done an annual physical on him, including a rectal, and one year I diagnosed a tumor in his prostate no bigger than this. [Dr. Williams wiggled the tip of his forefinger.] The leading urologist at Johns Hopkins agreed with the diagnosis and performed a prostectomy but was unable to take out all of the cancer. A year and a half later, he was walking and fell down suddenly. The tumor had metastasized to his leg—it had to be cut off at the hip. As time went on, he developed more pain; it become more and more severe. Morphine wouldn't relieve it—nothing would relieve it. I talked it over with the family: my two brothers, two sisters, and my mother. We didn't mention anything about the cancer to the patient, because in those days it was the custom to almost never tell a patient about a diagnosis of cancer. My family agreed to the following plan. I would give my dad heavy doses of barbiturate to keep him sleeping most of the time, and I wouldn't turn him over in bed very much, so that his lungs would become congested and he would develop pneumonia. If he developed pneumonia, I wouldn't treat it, and eventually he would die. Well, this is exactly what happened. He died with a minimum of pain, and I listened to his last heartbeat. Neither I nor any of my family has ever regretted what I did.

Dr. Williams's secretary came in, apologizing, and handed him a note on a small piece of paper. He read it and slapped his desktop lightly. "I have to go now and talk with this fellow who wants to get a teaching job here. I want to find out what he's like. I hope I've given you some insight into the character of R.H. Williams. My main trouble is that the day is not long enough to do all the things that I'm interested in." He rose to go. "I love solving problems, and through medicine I've discovered that everything in life is simple if you get off your tail and do something about it."

Then he was in motion, shaking my hand firmly and walking swiftly from the room, leaving me alone with the plaques, the photographs, the journal articles, the textbooks, and the webs of logic connecting body and mind that he had woven for me. Later I would read in one of his articles: "The ultimate supreme function of the body is mentation. Without mentation the body is not of significant use. Mentation plays the major role in all pleasures and pains. All abnormalities in mentation are associated with altered metabolism. . . ."

The day we talked was the last working day of Dr. Williams's life. Two days later, he was en route to Philadelphia by plane, hoping to assist in the solution of a baffling medical case. During the flight, he fell asleep listening to music on the stereo earphones. Somewhere between Seattle and Philadelphia, he suffered a final heart attack and never woke from that peaceful, airborne sleep.

The Social Element

THOMAS HOLMES, PSYCHIATRIST, RESEARCHER
IN PSYCHOSOMATIC MEDICINE

By the time of World War II, many of the potent antimicrobial drugs—penicillin, streptomycin, the sulfanamides—had come into common use. With ever more effective immunizations such as the Sabin and Salk vaccines, and with continuing improvements in infant nutrition and sanitation, infectious disease and infant mortality declined sharply in the postwar era.

As a result, the emphasis of medical research began to shift from infectious to chronic diseases. Here the battle lines were less clearly drawn. As Dr. Williams pointed out, diabetes, long considered a chronic, metabolic disease, may in fact be linked to an infectious virus. Yet, where are the causative agents for other chronic diseases such as cancer, emphysema, and cardiovascular disease? And why do people get sick when they do, contracting one disease rather than another?

For Dr. Thomas Holmes, searching for the answer to such baffling questions involves looking at the people who get sick rather than at the particular disease. During the course of a lifetime spent researching "psychosomatic medicine," he has become convinced that a person's environment and way of life have a profound effect on that person's health. This might seem like common sense; after all, who hasn't attributed a cold or a bout of flu to some event such as a period of overworking, the fatigue that results from travel, or similar emotional upsets? But such conclusions cannot be tested in a conventional clinical laboratory. And so, in order to document the "obvious," Dr. Holmes had to develop methods for studying people in their natural habitats, for viewing society itself as an experiment yielding information on the causative relationship between life-style and illness.

Dr. Holmes's interest in psychosomatic medicine began in the laboratory of Dr. Harold Wolff at Cornell. The starting point of this kind of research was the clinic and the psychobiologic orientation of Adolph Meyer, the famous psychiatrist who also influenced Robert Williams. Meyer was interested in the relationship of biology, psychology, and sociology to the processes of health and disease in man. In order to explore those relationships, Meyer created the "life chart," a device that organizes medical data in the form of a biography. Information is provided by the patient and is arranged by year and the patient's corresponding age. The entries on the life chart describe life situations: experiences having to do with growth, development, maturation, and aging, as well as the patient's emotional responses to each of those situations. Meyer listed separately the life experiences that are normally called "diseases," meaning a change in health status that could be medical, surgical, or psychiatric. In this way, the life chart allowed Meyer to research not only the occurrence of disease, but also the setting in which it develops.

Meyer's life chart was the foundation upon which Dr. Holmes built his own research. The culmination was the famous Social Readjustment Rating Scale (also known as the Holmes Scale), which quantifies the relationship of life experiences to disease. The SRRS has appeared in many contexts, from scientific colloquia to the pages of *Reader's Digest,* and is a cornerstone of current research in psychosomatic medicine.

When I visited Dr. Holmes's office one afternoon, the mail on his secretary's desk gave testimony to the wide-ranging impact of his work. There was a letter from an internist in Czechoslovakia, another from an anthropologist in Germany, one from a psychiatrist in South Africa, and one from a physical therapist in Omaha. The medical community, which had originally been skeptical of Holmes's approach, had come to accept his findings.

Dr. Holmes and I sat in his plant-filled office on the fifteenth floor of the medical teaching complex, and I asked him to look back over both his life and the development of psychosomatic medicine in this country. He leaned back in his comfortable chair and contemplated his coffee mug with a private smile. Then he began speaking in a calm southern drawl.

I wanted to be a doctor when I was four or five years old. I have vague recollections of discussing this with one of my aunts who was a schoolteacher. We used to sit for hours on the veranda of our old southern house in North Carolina. And ever since then, my professional life has been sequential, with each step leading to the next. I don't mean that this was due to prior planning, but I sure got where I was going. It came out of my approach to my life—a search for satisfaction, not happiness. Americans have hitched their wagons to a star ever since the Constitution let them pursue "happiness." You can only be happy in the future, but you can be satisfied every day.

I had three teachers who greatly influenced my life. The first was Miss Wiggins, who taught high-school English. She introduced me to Shakespeare, and as we were reading in class she would say, "All right, class, we will now skip over the next page and a half." Of course I'd go back later and look over those pages carefully. Miss Wiggins had a huge effect on my scholarly technique—my reading and writing.

The second teacher was a professor of philosophy at the University of North Carolina. The credo of his course was something like *Pata rey*, an Indian phrase which he interpreted to mean "Everything changes." He just died recently. The woman who was taking care of him called me up, and she told me, "Dr. Bradshaw is having his first coffee break with Horace Williams [another professor of philosophy], Frank Graham [who was president of the university], and Jesus." Everything changes.

I became a maverick in medicine because of the third teacher in my life. This was Harold Wolff, whom I worked with as a resident in internal medicine. The project I went to talk to him about had to do with viral diseases of the nervous system. He said, "Come back and talk to me next week." So I came back the following week, and he said that he'd recently been studying a subject named Tom who had mucous membranes of the stomach exposed so that it was possible to study what went on in the stomach directly. He said he'd also just finished a study on pain sensation in the nasal and paranasal spaces and had been impressed with what seemed to be similarities between the stomach mucous membrane and the nasal mucous membrane. "Why don't you look into that?" he asked. I thought; God, what is he talking about? And it was two months before I settled into looking into these problems.

I've been hooked on it ever since. That's when I started studying nasal function. I discovered a relationship between life situations, emotions, and nasal function. If you got angry over a given life situation, your nose got pale, dry, and shrunken. If you felt humiliated, helpless, unable to cope, your nose got red, wet, and swollen—all the symptoms of a cold. We would identify some of the feelings of helplessness and give some assessment of the intensity of that feeling, which let us quantify emotion in terms of nasal function.

This ultimately generated my first publications and my first book. No—I shouldn't say that—my first scientific publication was entitled "A Checklist of the Birds of Cape Martha." It was published when I was eighteen, before I had given up bird watching—an early love—for people watching. In retrospect, what I'm doing now is no different from what I did when I was bird watching. You know, I never made that analogy until just this moment. When you bird watch, you go into the field and you observe birds in their habitats, at four seasons of the year. You soon notice that in the spring and fall, there are lots of birds around, while in the winter and summer, there are hardly any. You become aware of geographical movements, of finite behavior, genetics, and the importance of environment. Bird watching had everything that wasn't taught in medical school, and my whole career in medicine has been taken up with proving scientifically in human beings what I had known all along from observing birds.

I guess what I'm saying is that you develop behavior patterns very early—competencies and skills. And no matter what you do, you will use these patterns.

Well, in the early days in Harold Wolff's laboratory, we used to say jokingly to each other that one could tell how a patient feels by looking at his nose or looking at the mucous membrane of the large intestine or measuring the skin temperature, implying that even early on, one could see predictable relationships. Given a certain emotion, you would predict the body change; given a certain body change, you would predict the emotion. It became a kind of in-house game. These were the early experiments in what is now called the "new etiology." We would go into the laboratory, measure a given organ function, then introduce a life situation—a caricature was a visit from the mother-in-law—then monitor the organ system and actually document the genesis of disease. Now, that's prospective research. We also did longitudinal studies, where we recorded what went on in the life situation each day—feeling states, behavior—and watch what happened to a given organ system. My good friend Dr. David Graham used to monitor my colon every day. I used to monitor his nose every day. As far as I know, I'm the only fellow in the history of medical science to be proctoscoped in the upright position.

Every day we had good results. There was very prompt feedback on these types of experiments. These were stimulus-response experiments in the true sense of the word—just like any good physiologist does in the laboratory. We were producing disease for the first time. The only people who had tried to do this before were the Germans in World War II. They subjected Jews to all sorts of terrible environments and observed what went on in the bodies of the Jews. We used to gasp as we read this stuff. (It got published during the war.) We were horrified at the inhumanity. But it was also poor science—the experiments weren't well designed.

Our experiments had all of the ingredients of prospective studies, identifying salient causative agents. This is the way we discovered mother-in-law as a pathogen and identified the father-in-law as a saprophyte, but not a pathogen [chuckles]. At that time, in the late 1940s, we were the outlaws of medical research. My good friend Larry Hinkle—a converted surgeon, thank God—gave his first paper at a society called the Young Turks, a society for young people getting into research. His paper talked about the relationship of events, emotions, and diabetes. This included variations of urine acetone, blood glucose, blood-acetone levels, liver production of ketones . . . and the past president of the society got up and said, "My God, is nothing sacred?"

We were contemptuous of those people because they didn't have the true message, you see, and we obviously did. It was kind of fun that way. The field of psychosomatic medicine was wide open to easy discovery, and you just couldn't have a project without striking gold. Much later, we discovered the writings of clinical scientists in the 1920s—beautiful clinical observations about the role of depression in diabetes, of the behavior that was observed, that sort of thing. In those days, they wrote down on paper what we learned only by word of mouth or by our own discovery. None of this beautiful stuff was in my medical textbooks.

The next step in the progression was when I came out here to work. At that point I had become interested in muscle physiology and muscle function and the disease of backache. I also knew something about colds and hay fever and aspirin. My first job out here was as psychiatric consultant to the tuberculosis hospital. I began applying the approach I had learned at Harold Wolff's lab, thereby making my consultation service a research activity. It became obvious that when you looked at the time of onset of tuberculosis in terms of what was going on in the life situation, the onset of disease coincided with a life crisis. The standard cliché of the hospital staff was that "it was in this setting that tuberculosis developed." But no one else had formally set down a reason for why a patient comes in with tuberculosis at age fifty-five, and the germ has been in his lungs since age forty.

At about that time, I began working with Dr. Loren Carlson, who was a professor of physiology. I was still studying muscle tension, muscle blood flow, and the mechanisms of muscle pain, and Dr. Carlson was very generous with his facilities and equipment. I was constructing small thermocouple needles that measured muscle temperature and blood gases. Dr. Carlson, an interesting fellow, was studying cold acclimatization, and one of the variables he was interested in was muscle temperature. The other dimension he was looking at was adrenal-cortex activity. Metabolism as a field was coming of age. The adrenal cortex was getting ready to replace the cerebral cortex [laughs]. Anyway, Dr. Carlson was working for the Air Force, and his grant came out of Alaska. He used to go up to Alaska in the wintertime and sleep out in forty-degrees-below-zero weather with thermocouples in his legs and back.

What we found in the preliminary experiments was a striking relationship between exercise and feeling states, between behavior and seventeen-ketosteroid production. We then wanted to control body activity to get a better relationship between emotions, feeling states, and steroid production. Since I was working at the tuberculosis hospital, I had 1,200 subjects flat on their backs—a beautiful way to control for behavior. So we decided to follow seventeen-ketosteroid excretion in these bedridden patients, and out of casual interest we also monitored changes in their chest X rays. It turned out, they were related! This was before cortisol and all the "wonder steroids" had been discovered or understood. Then we did systematic studies of behavior and life situations, and steroid excretion, and the natural history of tuberculosis, and it just fit together like a jigsaw puzzle.

It was obvious from the patients' life histories that many were divorcees, people who never married, alcoholics, peripatetic bums, jailbirds—the social element was caricatured. We were dealing with marginal people, which made the problem easier to study, since these people were at least two-and-one-half standard deviations from any cultural norm you cared to establish. At that point I hired a sociology graduate student, who introduced me to the questionnaire techniques of doing research. We began to systematize and quantify the social dimension. This early research was the beginning of the Schedule of Recent Experience (SRE), a questionnaire designed to elicit the sort of biographical information which Meyer used in his life chart.

By this time, tuberculosis was the disease of the Skid Row, the state mental hospitals, and the state penitentiary. We saw one population giving rise to all three of these diseases: crime, tuberculosis, and schizophrenia. When we looked at the incidence of these things among patients in the TB hospital, there they were. Many of them had criminal records, and at least 25 percent were schizophrenic. This put psychiatry, medicine, and sociology together.

Then we said, "What about tuberculosis in the community?" We studied the demography of tuberculosis by dividing the city up into socioeconomic areas, and used the area of residence as an index of life-style. We found striking relationships between area of residence and the morbidity of tuberculosis. It was a Skid Row disease, a city-center disease. So now we had documented the psychology, the physiology, and the sociology, and this is what my original mentor had suggested all along.

From tuberculosis it was an easy series of steps to apply the same approach to other diseases. We analyzed some 5,000 case histories of patients with cancer, with ulcers, with schizophrenic symptoms; a wide variety of diseases. As we did with tuberculosis, we went through the patients' life charts, picking out the life-change events present in their lives at the time of onset of disease. We then compiled a list of forty-three life events empirically observed to occur just prior to disease onset—marriage, trouble with the boss, jail term, death of spouse, change in sleeping hapits, retirement, death in the family, a vacation, and so on.

The SRE is based on the importance of those forty-three events. It is a questionnaire which asks the respondent whether each of those forty-three events has occurred in the last twelve months, and if so, how many times. Here are some typical questions from the questionnaire [he read from a paper on his desk]: "During the last twelve months, have you had a lot more or a lot less trouble with the boss? a major change in sleeping habits?" And so on down the list of forty-three events.

The onset of a patient's symptoms could almost always be tied to a crisis in their life situation. There was no—there still isn't any—other explanation for why people get sick when they do.

So, once I had mastered tuberculosis, it was easy to understand the other diseases. I was told in my medical-school pathology course that if one could understand cancer, inflammation, and tuberculosis, one would know all that was worth knowing about medicine. It took me thirty years to realize that was a very, very true statement.

The result of all of these case studies was the Social Readjustment Rating Scale (SRRS). The scale shows the *amount* of change implied by each of the forty-three life events in the SRE which seemed to be tied to disease. For example, the death of a spouse is the most important possible life event and is worth 100 Life Change Units on the SRRS. Divorce is worth 73 units, a jail term is worth 63 units, marriage is 50 units worth of life change, and so on down to Christmas, with 12, and being caught jaywalking, which is only worth 11 Life Change Units.

The SRRS gave us a unique tool to arrive at quantitative definitions of life crises and how they related to disease. The relative importance of each item is determined not by the item's desirability, not by the emotions associated with the item, not by the meaning of the item for the individual. It is the *amount of change* that we are talking about, and how it empirically relates to the onset of illness.

Using the SRRS to score the SRE has great predictive abilities. Based on retrospective studies, we were able to determine that if a person accumulates more than 300 Life Change Units over a twelve-month period, that person has an 80 percent chance of becoming significantly ill at some point in the near future. Those with 150 to 299 Life Change Units have a 50 percent chance of getting sick in the near future, and with less than 150 units one has only a 30 percent chance of getting sick soon.

Of course, the other question is why a certain person should get disease A rather than disease B. Some people with 300 Life Change Units get cancer; others get hundreds of warts. In the trade, that difference is known as specificity. The Life Change magnitude on the SRE says, "This is the time you will get sick." But one's perceptions of the life-change event and its significance account for the type of disease which occurs. The specificity theory is based on the field of psychodynamics. The coping mechanisms you have learned in life determine how you react to a specific life situation. If your style is to attempt to shut it out, you're apt to get colds, hay fever, and asthma. If your style is to run away from problems, you may get diseases like backache, rheumatoid arthritis, and osteoarthritis. If your style is to get angry and to want to get even with the situation, you're going to get a peptic ulcer. If you just want to get it over with, you're apt to get diarrhea. But that is not my work as much as it is Dr. David Graham's, who was also in Dr. Wolff's laboratory.

By the time we had all of this worked out, the public was ready to hear it. Alvin Toffler wrote me up in his book *Future Shock*, and I made some television appearances, which brought a huge public response. This gave me the chance to try an experiment in widespread prevention. On national television, I outlined a set of simple instructions for coping with life change, for realizing that one pays a price for life change. Here are the instructions [he read from a paper]: "Become familiar with the life events on the scale and the amount of change they require. Put the scale where you and the family can see it easily several times a day. With practice you can recognize when a life event happens. Think about the meaning of the event for you and try to identify some of the feelings you experience. Think about the different ways you might best adjust to the event. Take your time in arriving at decisions. Anticipate life changes and plan for them well in advance if possible. Pace yourself. It can be done even if you are in a hurry. Look at the accomplishment of a task as a part of daily living and avoid looking at such an achievement as a 'stopping point' or a time for letting down. Remember, the more change you have, the more likely you are to get sick. So, the higher your life-change score, the harder you should work to stay well."

I wasn't saying that one needs to be bored and uninteresting to be healthy. I was advocating stability, not monotony—stability and creativity.

The requests for copies of these instructions poured in. We sent them out with questionnaires to assess results.

The response to this attempt at primary intervention was a 20 percent reduction in disease for the following year among those people who received our questionnaires and followed those simple instructions.

The reaction of the medical profession was quite different. Doctors had moved away from the reductionism of the fifties, and their attitude toward me was "So what else is new? We've known this all the time!" Of course, the surgeons continue to ignore the whole thing. But in the fifties, when we were starting our research, our beliefs were restricted to the American Psychosomatic Society. This was composed of internists, pediatricians, a few obstetricians and gynecologists, not too many psychiatrists and public-health doctors, and almost no surgeons.

So now the medical establishment is waking up, and I am also able to work directly with the public and with my own patients. Oh yes, I still work on the individual level. I'm a doctor, and I've got to keep my skills as a doctor sharp. Along the way, this has contributed to my income, which is another benefit, but not too much and not too often. Some of the patients I see don't pay me. Psychoanalysts used to say that if the patient didn't pay, he wouldn't get better. But I've tested that hypothesis empirically. As a matter of fact, one way to get people better is to stop charging them.

When I'm working with individual patients, I tailor my techniques to that particular patient's needs and expectations. With some patients I spend time reassuring them, giving them emotional support, letting them ventilate their feelings, letting them flirt with me, if that's what they want to do. Sometimes I share any insight I might have about what seems to be going on in that patient's life. What all this does is quiet the patient down and allow him to learn about what he is doing with his life, and how he might modify his behavior. This can mean how he might cope with a job change, or with getting married—whatever in his life is going to require an adjustment.

It all depends on what they expect from me. If they expect me to act like a "real" doctor, if they've come to see me just to get a pill, I'll spend some time with them, tell them what I think is wrong, and then give them an appropriate prescription. I'll tell them that this pill is apt to work, and 80 percent of the time it does. I have great respect for the physiological effect of the placebo and for the therapeutic powers of suggestion. But as I say, my techniques vary from patient to patient. Some think that what I should do is analyze dreams, so we spend most of our time analyzing dreams. This works about as well as somebody else's pink pills.

If you think back now, the whole history of what I've been telling you involves the patient as the point of departure. The patient will come in and say, "Every time my mother-in-law comes, I get asthma." So the clinic generates the question, and then you go into the laboratory to test it. When we studied the demography of tuberculosis, we used the city of Seattle as a laboratory. We just moved from the hospital to the community and applied the same laboratory techniques. We've really never left the experimental model, and all along the experimental questions have come out of patient care. By the way, we also became interested in what is effective treatment— why some patients recovered from tuberculosis and others did not. We found that it was tied to assets—what the patient had going for him in terms of psychological and social stability. If you had TB and you were married, the probability was that you'd get better. If you weren't married, you probably wouldn't get better. Now what is it that the doctor does that may or may not influence outcome?

Well, in order to study that, I have to treat patients. But when I'm working with them, I never talk about my "theories." I never even use the word theory—do you think that I have one? [Laughs] Psychologists use the word all the time—it has some magical meaning for them. But I never really wondered whether I had a theory or not. Some people say I do and some say "No, it's all just common sense." With my patients I avoid the whole issue. I tell them what the facts are, how I got the facts, and what I think they need as a patient.

You see, what I'm advocating is a diversified approach to both diagnosis and treatment. The doctor-patient relationship gives this approach a cohesiveness, purpose, and direction for the patient. Anything I do to or for a patient, either directly or as a result of my "orders," serves as a symbol which constantly reassures the patient of my continuing interest and support, which helps make the patient feel more secure. And that's the most important result. In our society, which is undergoing rapid change, individuals often experience considerable difficulty finding their place in life. So, many of the illnesses experienced by man may occur as a by-product of attempts at adaptation. For me, being a good doctor means helping people adapt.

The Significance
of Tools

LOUIS DICARO, KIDNEY-TRANSPLANT SURGEON

Deep within the university hospital, the sign on the formidable gray doors read "Operating Rooms: Authorized Personnel Only." Beyond was a shuffleboard-court-length stretch of shining linoleum leading up to a wide yellow stripe beside the nursing station. "All persons past this line must wear scrub attire," read another sign. There was a washable scoreboard on the wall to schedule the day's events. Next to Room #8 a nurse had written: "Renal Transplant: Longfeather/ Surgeon: DiCaro."

Louis DiCaro, dressed in the light blues of a surgeon's scrub suit, crossed the yellow stripe and paused beside the nursing station. He was a researcher who made the operating room his laboratory. He was gazing downward, burying his chin in the crease of his dangling surgical mask. His mouth worked a piece of gum in a steady, powerful rhythm. Stocky and middle-aged, DiCaro moved in the manner of a boxer or a wrestler. His scrubs fit naturally—a set of dignified pajamas.

Past the nursing station was one more short stretch of hallway, ending in a wall decked with sinks and soap dispensers. DiCaro looked up at the door to Room #8, opening onto the hall from the left, then at the door to #7 directly across from it. He scowled and bit down on his gum. Things were off to a bad start this morning.

It was not the fault of the surgeon in #7, DiCaro's partner on the transplant team. He had been working since eight o'clock on the kidney donor and had now exposed the kidney without difficulty. It was ten o'clock, time for the transplant to take place. The problem was the plastic surgery going on in Room #8. Inexplicably, it was taking longer than expected and tying up the room DiCaro needed for the transplant recipient, Donna Longfeather.

The act of transplantation—removing a kidney from one body and grafting it inside the body of a recipient whose own two kidneys have ceased to function—was for DiCaro only an intermediate step in a meticulous sequence of events. For several days he had supervised the preparation of the recipient, an American Indian woman in her fifties. Heavy doses of immuno-suppressive agents had made it more likely that Donna Longfeather would accept the foreign tissue, and DiCaro's assistants had inserted a catheter deep into her venous system to record the condition of her heart during the surgery. Now she lay waiting on a gurney beyond the nursing station, supine on a milk white sheepskin blanket that she preferred to the hospital linen. A serious disease had damaged her kidneys beyond repair, and now her fate lay between a lifetime of costly and difficult dialysis treatment or the chance of a successful renal transplant. She had come more than a thousand miles to be operated on by DiCaro.

The donor had been chosen with equal care. Most living kidney donors are related to the recipient because of the greater chance of tissue compatibility among relatives. The woman lying on her side with her healthy kidney exposed in Room #7 was Donna's twenty-five-year-old daughter. DiCaro had subjected her to a battery of medical tests to be sure that she was in perfect health. He also took care that she was willing to be a donor, since he strongly believed that if the donor was the slightest bit reluctant, or if there were any underlying psychological problems, the best course was to "find" a medical reason to exclude that person as a donor.

Strict adherence to a protocol had made renal transplantation a reasonably optimistic operation, an experiment that bore a high degree of repeatability. DiCaro had been one of the first surgeons in the world to transplant kidneys, and the techniques he helped developed were now being used by more than 200 surgical teams around the world. Even now, he had performed more transplants than almost any other living surgeon. His high percentage of success attested to his idea of perfection of technique as a means of controlling variables.

DiCaro studied a spot on the floor for a few more moments, then turned and walked back past the nursing station toward the bed where Donna Longfeather lay. He spoke a few words to her and checked the placement of the catheter and IV tubes. DiCaro was well known for the personal attention he gave every one of his transplant patients, from the time he accepted their case he became their primary physician. He didn't want other doctors meddling with them without his consent. Each patient was an integral part of his research efforts, another potentially successful case, and DiCaro felt that continuing vigilance was the best way of preventing complications.

The surgeon in #7 was losing his temper. Classical music emanating softly from a radio propped on a stool in one corner no longer soothed him. "This is ridiculous, having to wait for a plastic surgery," he complained to the nurses and the surgical resident who were helping him. "I don't want to poison this woman for an extra hour." He was referring to the anesthesia being administered by a silent anesthesiologist standing amid a mass of tubes and wires at the head of the operating table. The surgeon passed his hand lightly over the surface of the exposed, pinkish kidney, then with a sigh removed the shiny metal retractors from the incision and let it close, piling some sterile towels over the opening. He gave the towels a light pat and stared at the ceiling. "Is there a sterile chess set anywhere about?" he asked. A nurse laughed.

Minutes later, the plastic-surgery patient was wheeled out of #8, and technicians scrubbed the floors with disinfectant, readying the room for DiCaro. All the tools used by the plastic surgeon were taken off to be sterilized, and a new set was assembled. DiCaro was particular about instruments, preferring certain variations on the armamentarium of scalpels, forceps, needles, and sutures.

He stood at the sink, washing his hands and forearms with iodine soap, scrubbing and lathering longer than the required time. Then, with his mask drawn up over his mouth, he strode into Room #8 and let the sterile scrub nurse dress him in sterile surgeon's gown and gloves. Donna Longfeather was being prepped for the operation. Nurses had transferred her to the operating table and strapped her arms onto extension boards that kept them outstretched while she lay on her back. The extended arms gave the anesthesiologist ample room to start anesthesia and connect a bag filled with a unit of blood for transfusion in case Donna lost any of her own.

DiCaro took his position at the table with a surgical resident and intern across from him and a medical student helping out on his left. The nurse, a tall, impassive man with Scandinavian features, stood by at the foot of the table to pass instruments. DiCaro muttered for a scalpel and extended his gloved hand with the dark forearm hair matted in rows beneath the glove. The operation began.

The surgeon in Room #7 had reentered the body cavity of Donna's daughter. He began carefully ligating the vessels that attached the kidney—the large renal artery and vein, the ureter that snaked its way toward the bladder. It was essential both to ligate them well to prevent internal bleeding and to leave a sufficient length of vessel attached to the kidney for DiCaro to work with.

A few minor blood vessels began to bleed. The surgeon switched to the electric cauterizer, shaped like a thick pen and connected by wires to a power supply. The air sang from the hum of the voltage passing the cauterizer's tip and singeing shut the bleeding spots with a small puff of smoke. A smell rose, like human hair put to a match flame.

The door opened to DiCaro's kick, and he came in with hands held aloft and sterile. He bent over the donor, wanting to know how big the kidney was. The fist-shaped organ lay gleaming up at him from its bed of retroperitoneal fat. Several ribs had been cut away to allow the surgeon better access. DiCaro nodded and chewed his gum in movements barely visible through the mask. He returned to Room #8.

A nurse in #7 wheeled out a small table, placing it between the surgery and the door. With the careful movements of an acolyte she opened two packages of sterile towels and placed them neatly folded near a small stainless-steel basin and several instruments, forceps, and scalpel. She positioned an overhead lamp to give direct illumination and set an IV bag on an adjacent rack with the long IV tube leading down to the metal basin.

The surgeon made a few final movements, the final disengagements. As the severed ureter squirted urine for a few moments, he joked at the way it was "peeing all over the place" but added in a more serious tone that this was a good sign. With a continuous motion he lifted the kidney out and, turning, placed it carefully on the sterile cloths on the small table.

DiCaro materialized, eyes intent on the table and its center, where the healthy, flesh-colored organ glistened roundly, a few bedraggled vessels running out from its indented hilus. He bent over it, touched it appraisingly. It had become his kidney, his medium. He trimmed off several tiny veins that could cause hemorrhage, and cut the ends of the larger vessels square to ease the process of sewing. With the plastic IV tube he began to perfuse the kidney, coaxing fluid into the artery and through the unseen complexities of glomeruli, tubules, and ducts, his gloved thumb cautiously milking the tissue until drops of clear fluid fell from the renal vein and ureter. His grip gained familiarity until he was not asking whether this kidney would be accepted by the woman lying in #8, but he was asserting with the quiet confidence of movements repeated over thousands of operations that yes, the operation would work.

Now he was satisfied. Straightening up, with the kidney cupped in one broad hand, he walked to the door, ignoring the trickles of fluid from the flaccid vessel endings. He disappeared into #8.

In #8 there was no classical music, no humor. The initial delay had made DiCaro even more businesslike. Placing the kidney on a flat portion of Donna's abdomen, he made furious preparations for its interment, delving with an electric cauterizer deep into the body cavity. The preferred technique of renal transplantation involved leaving the host's own kidneys intact if possible, and placing the new one in a lower location just above the pelvis.

On the other side of the cloth draped at the head of the operating table to demarcate the sterile zone, an anesthesiologist adjusted fluid levels, checked blood pressure and respiratory status of the unconscious patient, and now and then peeked over the cloth to watch the operation from his nonsterile vantage point.

DiCaro carefully slid the kidney into the opening. In a low voice he asked for needle and sutures, and within seconds his hands were darting up and down, probing the needle through delicate vascular walls, letting the resident clamp the needle from the other end and draw it through, then tying a series of knots, rapid as bee stings, and finally moving his hands slightly to the side for the resident to snip off the loose ends. Several times he looked up impatiently at the nurse, who was having trouble threading the needles quickly enough.

"Do you want me to add more blood?" the anesthesiologist asked. Donna had been losing a small amount steadily for the past five minutes.

"What kind of question is that?" snapped DiCaro from the corner of his mask, not looking up from his work. "What do you think? And what about the mannitol and the Laesix, are they going in?"

"I'll get on it right now," promised the anesthesiologist, whose attending had just walked into the room.

"Hey, Bill." DiCaro had somehow noticed the entrance of the senior anesthesiologist. "How many years have we been doing this operation?"

"Twelve years."

"That's twelve times 365 days, isn't it, Bill. Now we've worked out a certain protocol, haven't we?" DiCaro's stitching movements punctuated his words. "We *always* use blood and mannitol and Laesix, and I want to know why your man has to wait for me to ask him."

The attending apologized for his student.

"By God, this better not happen again, Bill. If this kidney goes sour . . ." He leaned more intently over the surgical field, sewing the renal artery onto the external iliac artery, a high-pressure cord of blood. As he made the connection, little jets of blood squirted up past his fingers, flecking the wrist of his gloves. "Give me suction," he said, louder than usual, moving his hands faster as the air in the room seemed to thicken.

One by one, the problems resolved. The kidney was securely in place. DiCaro paused to point out some structures to the medical student holding a large spatulate retractor, and to the intern whose retractor had been keeping the loops of bowel out of DiCaro's way for the past two hours. DiCaro checked the kidney's attachments one final time while the nurse counted sponges to make sure all were accounted for. Layer by layer DiCaro drew the tissue back over the kidney, sewing muscles together with syncopated movements. At last there was no more need for retractors, and only Donna Longfeather's bronze skin remained cleaved. Patiently working his way along the crescent of incision, DiCaro and the resident pricked and pulled, knotted and snipped, until there was only a raised line of flesh, which he patted down with the tip of his forefinger, the finishing motions of a master craftsman. The medical student beside him breathed a deep sigh.

Everyone stretched. Scrub had been broken. The operation was over. The chances for success were good, but DiCaro wasn't pleased. "Most operations," he grumbled, "are a lot more fun than that." He walked past the anesthesiologist, who was beginning to wean Donna from sleep, and picked up the clipboard with the anesthesiologist's chart of the surgery. He glowered over it while the resident and nurses unstrapped the patient from her crucified position.

"Can you hear me, Mrs. Longfeather?" asked the anesthesiologist. The dark eyelids trembled. Donna's gurney had been wheeled in, complete with the sheepskin blanket. Someone had already gone to inform the family waiting upstairs that all had gone smoothly despite the delay. DiCaro walked back to the operating table. Putting his hands underneath the patient, he called out, "One, two, three," and with the help of the resident, intern, and nurse lifted her back onto her bed.

Technicians returned to prepare the room for the next surgery. DiCaro dropped his mask and joked with one of them, beginning to shed his hard, driving solemnity.

Watching him, I thought back to another morning when he had paced around his office, smoking a cigarette like the tough guy in a Western, his sleeves rolled up. He had wanted to do "some philosophical explaining" of the way he approached medicine and research.

Most of us have a fairly general idea of what we'd like to do, and then circumstances more less mold what we actually do. When I got into medical school I was interested in internal medicine, but I worked with some surgeons one summer who were taking care of patients with tuberculosis. In those days tuberculosis was a terrible disease—people spent two or three years in a hospital, flat on their backs. But they were cured by the surgery, which greatly impressed me. It was avant garde surgery with a degree of danger, and it appealed to my personality, because I liked problems which could be solved.

That led me into becoming a surgical house officer, and at that time both vascular surgery and cardiac surgery were new. I was very interested in cardiac surgery, and probably would have become a heart surgeon, but the opportunity for that was quite circumscribed when I finished my residency, and at that time transplantation was opening up as a field, so I got into that.

At that time, we had a lot of problems in transplant surgery which were seemingly unsolvable. The surgical technique had been worked out. It was a vascular surgical technique not all that different from fixing, say, an artery, but the biological problems were terrific. We had many problems that we couldn't anticipate. So it was something new, and it required a great deal of personal physical input. It was basically a challenge, a real challenge of everything I had ever learned—not just my surgical skills, but also all of the medicine that I'd known and a lot I didn't know.

The field has given me an opportunity to develop something with huge therapeutic potential, which has not yet been fully realized. Transplants have made a tremendous impact in the twenty years since I started, but nowhere near the impact they will make. Now, whether it will always be a surgical procedure such as we know now, or whether it will involve cell transfers to compensate for endocrine deficiencies, is a question only time will answer. Then, too, there is the chance that transplantation could be expanded to include the implantation of artificial organs, in terms of those organs which could be copied by artificial devices. The heart certainly is an example of this. As far as we know it's a pump and only a pump. The lung, on the other hand, is a membrane for gas exchange, but there are certain peculiarities of the lung which may represent other functions which are not yet worked out: detoxification and so on.

There's no question that we've extended life considerably for those people who have received kidney transplants, and the successful recipients have gone on to lead very useful lives. The longest-lived transplants I've got are some allografts from nonidentical twins in 1959. I've got quite a few from the early sixties still functional, and also quite a few that were done when I first came here, in 1968.

It's a common fiction that in a field like this you get explosions of achievements, and the whole thing races away to utopia. Things don't really happen like that. In vascular surgery the original work was done on blood-vessel suturing back in the early part of the century, but only a few people were successful at it, and that's because they were supermeticulous. The field's development had to wait for a lot of advances in other, unrelated areas: anticoagulants had to be developed, antibiotics, better anesthetics, better understanding of asepsis, prosthetic devices. All those things took many years. Cardiac-surgery people were doing valvular operations back in the early part of the century, but they failed because they didn't have blood transfusions or anticoagulation, asepsis was poor, and anesthesia was often nonexistent. Now, transplantation, as I said, has other problems. We simply don't understand why grafts work. We talk about it, we have theories, we have experiments to support the theories. The simple truth of the matter is *we don't know why they work*. The theories simply don't explain in particular why an operation that *shouldn't* work according to theory does in fact work.

In principle, all grafts should be rejected because they're foreign to the host. The Burnett theory of immunologic surveillance means that the body should reject everything that is nonself. And it doesn't happen. We don't know whether the drugs we use modify the reaction, and if they do, how. There's a lot of knowledge which is not yet available, and it's anyone's guess how we'll come to solve the problem. We could come at it through histocompatibility studies, or better blood therapy, or perhaps better immunosuppressive maneuvers. It's very possible that we'll come at it through a better understanding of what it takes to persuade the body to accept foreign substances. That's a more complex problem than any of the ones we're working on. We don't have the technology to explore that yet.

There's a book up there [he pointed to the bookshelf behind him] called *Immunology for Students in Medicine,* by Humphrey and White, and in the preface of that book the authors point out that some people like to look down their nose at technology, saying that technology is a mere application of all these marvelous ideas. But if it weren't for the technology that became available for immunologists, they'd still be titrating serum. *Technology* is what opened up the field of immunology: the availability of the special apparatus to separate out various coagulants, the equilibrant gels with which you can do electrophoresis. One cannot casually dismiss the significance of tools.

Until the engineers developed radiotelescopes, the physicists had no idea of the existence of quasars and pulsars and black holes. They had to have the technology to be able to find them. And I suspect that the tools to enable us to find the answers to some of the problems of transplantation have not yet been forged. Take pregnancy. That's a very profound problem. If the placenta is a foreign growth, why isn't it rejected until just the right time? And why aren't tumors rejected by the body? Nobody knows, but you could come up with a variety of concepts which, given the right tools, could be studied. One of them would be that the host lays down a film, if you will, over the antigens of the tumor or graft or placenta, and that film protects it from rejection. But the problem is that we don't yet have the right tools, because these problems have to be studied not *ex vivo* but *in vivo,* as far as we know.

Doctors are people; and like anybody else, if you've got a going concern you'd like to keep it going in the direction you think it ought to go. It isn't necessarily where it should go, because we don't have 360-degree vision, we simply don't. We had a great time in this country for about fifteen or twenty years, when most everybody thought biomedical research was the greatest thing in the world. We let ourselves get caught in giving interviews to people like *Medical World News* and that kind of magazine, and it was a miracle a minute in those days.

Unfortunately, a lot of it was rhetoric. The promised fruits failed to materialize. I'm one of the people who participated in that phase from about '62 to '70. In 1970 the rhetoric began to slow down, but for five or six years, transplantation was the darling of surgery, and there were a lot of people who went off the deep end.

They—it was the golden age. Everyone was so flushed with the success of what was literally thought to be impossible five or ten years before that they thought all things were possible. Unfortunately, it led surgeons to do things that damn near discredited transplantation. The biggest single contribution to that lessening of enthusiasm was cardiac transplantation. All the entrepreneurs rushed in, and they were doing heart transplants two and three a day in some places, and of course patients were dropping like flies, and the only way the surgeons could keep up their press relations was to do more. So they diluted off the deaths, but ultimately that's a losing game—everything goes "whump."

There were enormously bad reverberations from all this, lots of bad publicity, and it seriously impaired transplantation on virtually every scene. I don't mean patients were more cautious. Since people who are dying with a disease are desperate, they will do anything. They go to all kinds of quacks, for example, so if you wanted to you could easily get people to come. But it turned off the responsible members of the profession, and the public agencies that fund these things and are charged with overseeing them got very disenchanted, because really it was a farce.

The same thing happened with liver transplants. Other people got into the liver game, and they failed. They almost discredited liver transplants; they hadn't done the basic work. My co-worker and I used to do two liver transplants a day in dogs. It's just a lot of work; you don't realize how much work that is. We'd do two a day every damn day for months on end, and study them to our hearts' content. We perfected the technical aspects, which are quite difficult, much more difficult than a kidney transplant or a heart transplant. And we also perfected the means of giving the immunosuppression and deciding when the rejection was coming, for years—that stuff went on for years: Shumway, the pioneer of heart transplantation, spent a good ten years of his life working on heart transplants in dogs before he ever did a human case. Due to people like that there's been progress. When it's right, when it's all worked out, transplantation could be like a coronary bypass.

Once the technology of transplantation is sufficiently developed, every surgeon who possesses the fundamental surgical techniques will be able to do it. There are plenty of surgeons who can sew blood vessels. But the right combination hasn't arrived yet, and so at the present time transplantation is largely restricted to those like myself who have done a lot of work in the field, with a lot of experience not only with patients but with animal experiments.

These are people who have—not really intuition. That usually means something that comes out of the sky, but it is intuition in the sense that you have a background and you don't really have a logical process that tells you to do this or that, but you have a feel for it. And that's why people who haven't got the background shouldn't get into it now, because we haven't got all the rules laid out. The rules for an appendectomy are simple. You can teach a housewife how to diagnose appendicitis, and she'll be right about as often as an experienced surgeon.

The reason that people adopted this kind of reductionist approach to problems is that it's been fruitful in the past. Look at Pasteur and germ theory. It's simple, it's manageable, and it permits us to analyze rather than having to synthesize. It's just like the kid who takes a clock apart one day. He may understand how it works, but he can't put it back together. Well, that's just a natural bent in human beings.

Does the mental state of the patient affect the outcome of a surgery? I don't know. The answer to that is "I can always say no because I can't verify it, and I have no means of verifying it." But privately I have wondered about the psychology of life. You see some things which are just not so easy to explain in scientific terms. The problem is you can't count on it, you can't manipulate it. I have no illusions about the fact that psychology has played an important role in medicine, but we don't know how to manipulate it. I've been very, very uneasy about allowing it to dominate or even enter my thinking when I'm trying to take care of a patient. The best thing you can do for a human being or an experiment is to be as objective as you can, and it's hard to be objective. But it's very unwise for the person who has to make very difficult decisions every day to rely on any kind of magical thinking. If you do, you make terrible, terrible mistakes, of the kind that aren't necessary if you have the scientific principles to avoid them. We can't rely on magic. We're not witch doctors, we're not shamans.

At the same time, surgery's very superstitious. It's a very ritualized life. We do certain things in a certain way, and if it's not done that way, we'll get upset. We call it preparation or getting psyched up, or any one of those things, but it's a little like the ballplayer who chews gum and fusses with his hat—that's a magic ritual. We're perhaps a little more sophisticated about it, but I don't know. There could be somebody up in 4D looking down on us and laughing his head off. Basically, the things I do for an operation are that I plan as best I can, and always make bigger plans, anticipate more problems than I hope to encounter, try to get myself to a level where I anticipate trouble. If I have it I'm not trying to come up to that level, I'm already up there. It's easy to come down, but it's harder than hell to get up. It's a mistake to have an overly sunny attitude and have things turn out bad because you're not serious enough about the operation.

PART V

Personal Lives

The wounded surgeon plies the steel
That questions the distempered part;
Beneath the bleeding hands we feel
The sharp compassion of the healer's art
Resolving the enigma of the fever chart.

—T. S. Eliot, *East Coker*

A physician's personal life can be invisible in the diploma-hung office, the sterile hospital ward. Perhaps this is why the public image of a doctor's private world runs to extremes. The picture of material wealth and comfort, of social status and power, jars with the reports of unhappy marriages and frequent divorce, of the impossible struggle between domestic and professional responsibilities, of the high rates of drug addiction, alcoholism, and suicide.

Many doctors I interviewed talked for hours about their relationship to medicine without mentioning other, more emotional relationships—family, friends, or simply time spent away from the medical sphere. So I asked four doctors to talk more deeply about these matters.

They did so hesitantly, often at a sudden loss for words, and worried about the impact that divulging any secrets could have on their career. "None of this must get back to my patients or my colleagues," one doctor warned; "I can't afford for them to know this about me."

Matthew Steinberg was willing to talk about his marriage of thirty years and how it had been affected by his successful medical career. The fact that his wife is a noted performing artist rather than a traditional "doctor's wife" brought the issues into clearer focus as he tried, in his early fifties, to discover where he and his family had come since the time he entered medical school. His marriage survives, and in fact most physicians seem to have a divorce rate below the national average. A recent survey of 100 doctors in a midwestern county showed that most doctors gave their marriage favorable marks, with the practitioners who worked the longest hours being most pleased with their marital situation.

Someone to Come Home To

MATTHEW STEINBERG, PSYCHIATRIST,
HUSBAND FOR THIRTY YEARS

We talked late into the night, seated at the kitchen table of his comfortable house in the suburbs of Chicago. At one point his youngest son came in to say good-night, then padded off to bed. His other children had grown up and gone, and his wife was out at a rehearsal of the dance company she directed.

A well-groomed dog was visible through a doorway, asleep on a rug in the darkened living room. Its snores blended with the ticking of an antique clock.

Matthew Steinberg's entire body seemed to prickle with energy in the midst of this stillness. "I'm glib and I know it, and I could talk for hours about these things, but I want you to know the emotions behind my words." His elastic features contorted with emphasis, and he shook his glass full of whiskey and ice cubes.

As the night wore on, his rhythmic speech blended with the metronomic, far-off clock, his voice rising and falling with humor and sadness, telling the story of his marriage, of his career as a psychiatrist. "The two," he said, running a hand quickly through his short, thick hair, "are really inseparable."

Well, let's begin at the beginning. I met my wife, Ann, the September after I was graduated from college. My mother introduced us. One thing I was sure of at that point in my life, at age twenty-one, was that I'd never marry any girl my mother introduced me to. But that summer, Ann had had a very traumatic experience in the dance company she was with. She fell in love with a homosexual. So she was very upset. She was only eighteen, and she was staying with her aunt, who was a good friend of my mother's. I'd broken up with my girl friend at the end of college, so anyway my mother said, "You really ought to take Ann out and have a beer with her and straighten her out."

I hadn't gotten into medical school yet, and already I was being put into the role of the healer! My mother kept after me and finally one night she was at her friend's house and I had to pick her up, and Ann was in the same house, so my mother said, "Why don't you go upstairs and meet this girl, and if you like her you can ask her out for a beer, and if you don't you can just say how do you do, good-bye." So I walked upstairs, and there was this incredibly breathtaking titian redhead with her hair down to here, wearing a tight black sweater and long black skirt, which was the fashion of the day. I nearly fell over. She was talking on the phone, and when she got off we were introduced, and I said, "Hi, do you want to go out for a beer?" And so off we went. It was love at first sight—corny, but true.

We visited each other on weekends while I was in grad school in physiology and Ann was studying ballet in another city. Then, in my freshman year of medical school, we eloped. She was twenty-one and I had just turned twenty-four.

It was March of my freshman year, and my best friend in my class in med school gave me all the anatomy-lecture notes that I had missed by being away for two days. They were beautifully done, with multicolored drawings of the parts, and on the top of the front page it said "Big Wedding Present!" But even though we were married we couldn't live together, because we had decided right off that both of our careers were important, and so we stayed at our respective schools until June, when she was able to get a fellowship to come to Chicago, where I was in med school.

After that, we basically went through med school together. Now, for me, that was marvelous because she was a much better roommate than the guy I'd lived with my freshman year. It was a great comfort to have my wife there when I would crawl home from school. Ann, however, was having a hard time adjusting to the dance company in Chicago, and she needed a lot of support—it was her first professional job. How much support could I give her as a sophomore med student? I was going to med school nine to five, five and a half days a week—it was relentless, absolutely relentless. I was just ingesting and spitting back at very frequent intervals a huge amount of factual information. So I'd come home at night with a whole load of homework to do, and Ann would be going out to a rehearsal. We'd manage to have dinner together, and then when she came home at midnight if I could still be awake we could spend some time together. The next morning I'd be up at dawn because I had to be at med school by eight o'clock and she'd sleep in.

This wasn't an atypical picture at all: the guy grinding out this huge amount of work in school and his wife having a job, and then the woman would make dinner and both would sit down and then the guy would go and start studying. There was very little contact. If I went out to a movie I fell so far behind in my work instantly that I felt a lot of anxiety and guilt.

At the end of my sophomore year there was a big set of exams plus Part I of the National Boards. Ann was doing two performances a day at this point, and she was exhausted all day without being able to figure out why. One morning she got up and started to brush her teeth and got terribly nauseated and started to vomit. As the technician friend of mine in the lab said, "The frog didn't ovulate, it had a litter." So, lo and behold, on top of all these exams and everything, my wife was pregnant.

Danny was born in January of my junior year, when I was in the middle of clerkships. The baby was born very quickly. Within an hour or so in the middle of the night we had a baby, and the next morning I had to go out and go to my clerkship. At the end of the day a nice resident gave me time off and said I could go see my wife. So, you know, on that level it was all struggling upstream. Everything we wanted to do that was in any way humanistic or personal or would make it possible for us to maximally share the experience of having a child had to be done in spite of our environment rather than because of the environment. Ann wanted to nurse the baby, and the nurses were giving her a terrible time, so I signed my own wife and baby out AMA—against medical advice—less than forty-eight hours after the childbirth, as a junior med student. I do remember, though, that the OB was pretty supportive; he let me be in the room for the birth—probably my being a med student made it possible—and it was the first delivery I had ever seen.

We came home with our baby and struggled to keep a contact going, and this continued through our senior year. Notice that I keep saying "our" year, because we really feel that we both went to medical school, only I got the piece of paper at the end. I got through it all, and I got a super-good internship right there in Chicago—a straight pediatrics internship. That gave me the privilege of working every day, every other night, and every other weekend for a year.

You figure it out. I was working thirty-six hours out of every forty-eight, and that wasn't an unusually rough internship. Got paid $100 a month, which was par for the course. That's when Ann and I really got hit, because when I got home for twelve hours, more often than not I was dead on my feet, and even though I'm a very, very high-energy person, I needed some sleep. What do think happened to our ability to simply sit down and have any kind of sharing, of interpersonal contact in a relaxed way, not to even mention sexual contact? Plus trying to spend time with my eighteen-month-old baby—it was a nightmare, really, perhaps far more for Ann than for me, and I don't say this in a patronizing way. She still had her work—dancing eight performances a week, which meant six evenings a week. I, on the other hand, was in this incarcerated state with five good friends for interns. I had a support system, albeit under total pressure.

Ann got no nurturing in her work. It was highly competitive. She never knew where the next role was coming from, and whether she would even get to dance in the next production. In my internship, I knew that if I produced well I would at least get some recognition for it, I would have plenty of work to do, and I would have a job the next year and the year after. What did Ann have for a support system? She had a half-unconscious husband twelve hours out of every forty-eight. The whole situation got summed up one day when Ann was taking Danny for a walk. He was a toddler and they were walking along a shopping street. A butcher came out of his butcher shop with his long white coat on about a half a block away, and Danny yelled "Daddy!" and broke away from Ann and started to run down the street toward this man. And you talk about medical humor. . .

During my residency, we had no money, and no chance to see each other, so when I got my dinner break I'd call home, and Ann would dash over to the hospital to have supper with me, with the baby in tow, of course. As often as not I'd never make it through supper because I'd get an emergency call and I'd have to leave Ann behind with the baby in the hospital dining room, maybe with some wife of another resident.

The intern year, though it was probably one of the most educational years of my career, was unquestionably the nightmare year of my training. As much in love as my wife and I still were, she became involved in a love affair, with someone with whom she was working. She told me about it with great guilt and consternation and tears and the whole thing. Then it happened again that same year with another man. From my part I'm sure that had I had the opportunity in terms of sheer hours, it could easily have happened to me. The situation of internship is really akin to military combat, and it's been documented over and over again that in the face of imminent death there is a tremendous upsurge of sexuality in many people—a need for sexual contact. My interpretation of it is that there's a need in the face of something that negates life to reaffirm life, and what can reaffirm life more than being involved in a love affair? Woody Allen would make a joke out of it—the opposite of death is sex. And I don't have to go into the gory details of what all this did to my ego.

In a way it's a miracle to me that we don't have more extramarital affairs and divorces during doctors' residencies. You talk to residents and they say, "Oh boy, I'm almost finished, boy, I'm going to get out of here, I'm gonna start to live." Guess what. By the time they're third-, fourth-, fifth-, sixth-year residents, they're working every fifth night or maybe every tenth night. Lo and behold they get graduated from this incredibly prolonged training, and they get to be a practitioner. Now they can work every night. Even if they're in a group practice they'll be working some nights.

What was it like for me? Well, I ended up being boarded in psychiatry, and six months after I completed my final fellowship training I went into private practice. I proceeded to start doing private practice just the way I'd done a residency. I put myself on call twenty-four hours a day, seven days a week. I had a professional apartment, which meant that I had my office in my apartment. It was one of those great big old apartments in New York City, in Manhattan. I didn't even have a separate telephone line. Can you imagine? In the interest of saving money I let our home phone number be the number my patients would call. I had this great big beautiful professional apartment and no money and was scared shitless that I would go broke. With the help of some friends I built a bunch of walls and created doorways, so that the patients could walk into the front foyer, which I'd split in half. Each half was about ten by ten feet, and one half was my oldest child's study—by this time I had three children—while the other half was my waiting area.

When I was seeing patients, my family had to ride the service elevator with all the building's garbage. The service-elevator man was a nice old punchdrunk fighter who used to tell funny stories and loved the children. But basically my family was riding a garbage elevator and my patients were coming up on the main elevator, all in the name of minimizing my expenses.

I never said to the family, "Don't make noise while I'm seeing patients." On the contrary, I told them to just live their normal lives, and if some noise came through, not to worry, it would become part of the therapy. But it was still a constant pressure on my wife and children that Daddy was seeing patients. What this did to my marital relationship, neither I nor my wife realized until much later. It reinforced an angry, sticky kind of dependence between my wife and me, because the guilt and anger went both ways. I was feeling guilty about making my family live like this so the debts could be paid off.

When I would come out of the office at the end of the day, I walked straight into my house and straight into my family, with no decompression time, and full of whatever I was dealing with—all that toxic stuff that comes pouring out at you when you're a psychotherapist. I had to keep it all inside, because the constraints that any doctor feels about telling his family about his patients are stronger when you've got psychiatric patients.

We did this until we couldn't stand it anymore, and then we moved back here and I went into teaching, and I've been at it now for twelve years. It's interesting that I had this fantasy about having free time in academia. Little did I dream that medical academia is the most pressured, the most competitive situation that you could dream of getting into.

They did a poll of the faculty of our medical school and found that the average faculty member was working fifty-two scheduled hours a week. That means that you've gotta add close to 25 percent more to find what he actually works. That's your role model. I have a wonderful Scotch friend who says that everyone's entitled to go to hell in their own way, but you don't have a right to try and force somebody else to do the same thing! But of course we do in medicine all the time—the professors do it with the students, the attending staff does it with the house staff, and on and on.

You're not talking to any paragon of virtue in this thing. I am fifty-two years old and I am still desperately struggling to get control over my own functioning as a physician and teacher. I'm doing better, but my average work week is well upwards of fifty hours still. Along with everyone else in the system I essentially have a job description which can't be done by one person, so I pull time from my family, from recreation, and from other kinds of creative activities. What I'm saying is that my training intensified my inability to say the shortest word in the English language: "No."

I really love what I do, which is why I go on doing it. But there are days when I get up and know I have to give a lecture or become involved in a teaching conference or a seminar, and I feel like a goddamned trained seal, and I don't feel like doing the act that day. I just don't want to bark and roll that ball on my nose and have everybody go, "Yeaaa, look at him, he's so marvelous, we can't do that."

Once I get started, I'm always all right, but Jesus, I would really rather stay in bed, and I can't permit myself to do it. This is a terrible confession, but I don't think I've every played hooky from medicine one day in my life.

We have a stereotype that's been set up and reinforced within medicine, which is that there aren't enough doctors to go around, and all the people who get sick will die immediately if some intervention doesn't occur. Now that's statistically—it's massively—untrue, but we've all bought into it. The unspoken equation is that if I don't show up for work, a human being will die, and that makes it very easy to say, "Oh my god, I've gotta be at work." But a lawyer doesn't say that, and a plumber doesn't say, "If I don't show up and fix the heating plant, somebody's house will be cold and they'll freeze to death." And if a pilot doesn't feel well, somebody else will fly the plane. So as a physician you have a degree of isolation that is unique in the world, because even if you're working with other people, you have the ultimate responsibility for a patient's welfare, and you can't share that responsibility with others.

So what are the benefits? Well, it makes us feel needed, but that ain't the same as being loved. The doctor is being needed and he may be worshiped, the patient may even fall in love with him in an infatuated way—but that's one of the great sources of disappointment. You get needed all right, but in a very demanding kind of way, and you don't get loved. Why the hell should someone love you for taking away their pain? You oughta take away their pain, but why should they love you for it? It's like loving the guy who fixes your car's carburetor. And yet, I went through long periods of thinking that my career would provide a kind of nurturing and love that I'd been looking for all my life.

Maybe this explains why doctors are such desperate chronic accumulators of material goods. They're the biggest suckers in the world. They buy more Cadillacs, more gadgets of every description; they are the craziest losers in stock-market schemes and real-estate swindles. Why is it these intelligent, highly educated people are constantly getting into these get-rich-quick schemes when they are already rich? It's because they've never gotten the love they thought medicine was going to give them. You keep curing your patients, and people seem to be very grateful, but when it's all over, there's this empty feeling in the pit of your stomach.

Talking personally again, it's been a very humbling experience to find out how many things I could refuse to do in my career. And guess what, the students didn't fall apart, the patients didn't fall apart, nothing fell apart. It was a shock to find out that I was expendable, and that there have been many occasions when my wife was far less expendable than I was. We damn near blew ourselves out of the water as a couple, because of the feeling on her part that she never got enough support from me, which was true, that I couldn't put my money where my mouth was and say, "Yes, damn it all, your dancing is just as important as my doctoring." It's only in the last five years that we really have tried to share equally in the marriage, and not say, "Oh well, my work has to be more important than anything because I'm saving lives."

I don't blame medicine completely. Lots of us were workaholics before we ever got to med school. Certainly to get through med school you have to have a certain compulsiveness. But medicine takes a lot of time and a lot of energy, and the fact of the matter is that to this very day, at the moment we're sitting here talking, my wife and I are still struggling. I made a lunch date with my wife for two days from now, Friday, 'cause there's a new little restaurant that I wanted to take her to. Yesterday I got a call from the cochairman of the residency committee at the university—there's a terrible problem with a resident. The cochairman is in desperate need for a meeting Friday at noon with all these mucky-mucks because this resident is graduating and the training staff doesn't want to give her an unequivocal bill of health. Even though the person has been completely free of psychiatric care for two years, the person once had an acute psychotic episode. So they need my input, because it's my department, to allow this person to go on to her next job. So I say to the guy on the phone, "Hey, who's going to help me when my wife wants a divorce because I broke the first lunch date I've made with her in months?" Like most medical humor, it isn't funny at all. I go home and I tell my wife about this, and she gets mad. Well, I get mad because she didn't support me, and I sarcastically say, "Thanks for being so understanding." She shoots back at me, "Thank *you* for being so understanding."

So we made a breakfast date. I looked in my book and said, "Dammit all, we've got to make another date." So we're going to have breakfast on Friday, and I never would have thought to do that just a few years ago. It never would have occurred to me to have a breakfast date and come in late for work, meaning after eight-thirty. But I'm going to have to actively restrain myself like this for the rest of my career. One plunge into getting impressed with my own importance, one plunge into overactivity in my field—one drink and I am going to get drunk.

Women in Medicine

ELLEN SALZMAN, WOMEN'S-HEALTH PHYSICIAN

Dr. Ellen Salzman sat with the twelve women medical students, their chairs pulled into a circle. She was small but intense, the focus of their attention. She was talking about what this gathering of women could accomplish in the months to come. The students had organized this support group for women in medicine and asked Dr. Salzman to lead it.

Among the varied faces gazing expectantly, questioningly, at her and each other, Dr. Salzman seemed barely older than the rest. In her late thirties, she had retained the energy of an adolescent, talking rapidly, openly.

Leading this group of women into discussions of how medical school affected their hopes, their self-images, and their lovers and spouses was only the latest strangely logical step in a mottled medical career that had often taken her down unexplored paths. Always she had been able to draw on her talents—her warmth, humor, and quickness, her ability to be alternately firm and vulnerable.

Simply to go to medical school, as a woman in 1966, had not been easy, but later there had been opportunities more closely suited to her—a rotating medical internship followed by a year as a GP at a university health center. After that had come two years gaining a master's in public health, then a year as a clinical instructor in a medical-school department of gynecology, and several years running family-planning clinics and training nurse practitioners in family planning.

Now Dr. Salzman had returned to the university setting for more training, this time in psychiatry. She had wanted to deepen her counseling skills, to sharpen her perceptions of herself and of her place as a woman in medicine.

"When I began this psychiatry residency," she told me one afternoon—we were seated in a small room adjoining the inpatient psychiatry ward of the county hospital, and the door had closed with an authoritative sound suggesting heavy locks—"only four out of the seventeen new residents were women. I was feeling, 'Oh god, here I go again—almost as outnumbered as I was in medical school.' For the past five years I'd been seeing almost exclusively women patients at the family-planning clinics, except when I'd counsel couples, and my staff for the nurse-practitioner training program was all women. Occasionally a male would wander through, but nothing like this.

"As a woman doctor on the psych wards, I'll have patients who persist in thinking that I'm a nurse. After three weeks of being here, they'll ask me who their doctor is. It's almost always women patients—the ones who are skilled at manipulating male physicians into getting what they want, who are looking for drugs or something like that.

"If I was right out of medical school, still pretty unsure of my identity, of what I was doing here, this would upset me, but I'm past all that."

I asked Dr. Salzman to talk about how she had arrived at this point. She took a sip of coffee, adjusted her position slightly (she was half-curled into an easy chair), and stared briefly at the high ceiling. "Well, okay," she said, "let me start at the beginning."

My father was a physician, and though he died when I was five, I'm sure he had a lot to do with my initial decision to go into medicine. His things had been left around the house—his stethescope, his microscope.

And medicine was sort of a natural for me in one way—I always did well in science in school. But I grew up in a very middle-class Jewish Wisconsin community, where girls did not become doctors—they married doctors. You went to college only to find a husband, and God forbid you should graduate.

Priority Number One was marrying a doctor. Number Two was a lawyer, and dentists were maybe Number Three—you know, as long as they were professionals or made a lot of money. And I'm really not sure why I was different and how I overcame that social mold. I was one of thirteen girls who hung together from grade school through high school. All of us graduated from high school, but only two of us went on to college. The rest got married. And I have an older sister who got married and has four kids—sort of had them one after another.

So, initially, almost everybody actively discouraged me from thinking about medicine. I remember thinking in junior high, "Well, I'll be a dental hygienist," because I had an aunt who was a dental hygienist.

Then in high school there was one counselor, God save this guy, who encouraged me. I don't know why, but he was really good about making sure that I had the right courses, that I had a chance. He told me about a scholarship that two physicians in the community offered each year to a graduating senior who was interested in pre-med and medicine. These two physicians were a married couple, and the woman was a role model for me. I'd known her ever since I was a little kid; in fact, she was my GP, which was unusual back then, because I know so few older women physicians. There just weren't many. Anyway, I applied for that scholarship and won it, and that gave me a lot more impetus.

By the time I started college, I was 100 percent sure that I wanted to be a doctor. Not that I was getting any more encouragement for it. My family could have cared less. My mother said to me, "You can do whatever you want as long as you get married eventually." My friends and friends' mothers thought I was crazy. One person said to me, "If you go to medical school it will be too bad because nobody will marry you." Someone else said, "You're just planning to go to medical school because nobody will marry you, but you'd drop out right away, right?" I finally got to the point where I said, "Screw all you bastards—I'm going to do it and show you that I'm really serious about it."

College was difficult. I was in competition with five hundred other pre-meds, and I think there was only one other woman. My pre-med counselor was very discouraging. When I got a C in freshman English, he told me that was it, I'd never get into medical school. He told me to stop right away and go into another field.

I first applied to med school after three years of pre-med, hoping that I could get in without finishing my fourth year. Everybody thought that was a joke, and even though I got put on the alternate list of one school, I didn't get in anywhere and ended up going off for the summer to Europe, feeling pretty discouraged.

I came back the day before the deadline for finishing an application for medical school—for applying for the MCATs and everything. I had twenty-four hours to decide whether or not I was going to do it. I finally said, "I'm going to do it, but I'm not going to tell anyone." People had seemed delighted that I hadn't gotten in the previous year, as if they knew that I wasn't good enough, smart enough. So I reapplied for everything, took my MCATs again and did much better, and was feeling pretty hopeful. One day I was talking to an older physician in the community, who said to me, "You know, you're going to have a tough time getting in, because they don't like to take women." He said, "I want you to go talk to the associate dean for medical-student affairs and tell him that if you get accepted to medical school you won't drop out. I know that sounds crazy, but you've literally got to write it in blood that you won't drop out of medical school, because they have that expectation of every female."

I went up to the dean and did exactly what that doctor said. I told him, "I want you to know that if I get accepted I will not drop out. I promise I will practice medicine." And a week later, the day before Thanksgiving, I got accepted.

I lost a few friends that fourth year of college, after I got accepted. That fourth year it was me against thirty of my male pre-med friends, and it was real clear that by getting into medical school I was taking up a place that they felt belonged to one of them. Not many of them got into med school. One went off to a Mexican medical school, one went off to an Italian medical school, one to dental school, and one went to law school. He had been pretty funny as a pre-med because he fainted at the sight of blood, but his mother wanted him to be a doctor.

So I was really excited when I got accepted, but I couldn't find anybody else to get excited with. People had thought that I couldn't do it, and when I actually did get in, they thought it was sort of stupid. It wasn't an accomplishment, in a lot of people's eyes. I sometimes wonder why in spite of all these odds I did pursue it, because I had a lot of women friends who were as bright as, if not brighter than, I was who got discouraged early and went into nursing, or med tech, or dental hygiene.

The other thing about it was the assumptions people began to make about me. I'll never forget sitting on the steps of the college library with a guy I'd known for years who had applied five times to medical school, had been rejected five times, and each year would take a job and reapply. I had just been accepted, and he turned to me and said, "Gee, Ellen, you must be a lesbian if you want to go to medical school." Most people didn't seem to think I was queer as much as they thought I must be really smart. The assumption was that if you were a woman, you had to be smarter than all of the men in order to get into medical school.

I started medical school in 1966—it was before the real influx of women into medical schools. During the Second World War, women went to medical school because the men were off fighting the war. But from the late 1940s to the late 1960s, there were almost no women in medical school at all. When I started, the nationwide figure was about 5 percent. I was one of seven women in a class of 170 students. It was real bad.

I became close friends with one other woman. Thank God she was there, and we got into trouble constantly because we were different from all the other women. They were from very small towns in Wisconsin, were extremely conservative, didn't smoke or drink or swear; they didn't go out, they didn't do anything. We all lived together, believe it or not, in a medical-sorority house. It was cheap—who had money in those days? And it was convenient, not far from the medical school. But it was deadly. My friend and I finally got kicked out of the sorority for drinking beer after finals with two of our male classmates. The other women felt that one should work hard and study hard and become a good doctor. For them, men were extraneous. After that I didn't see very much of the other women. Everything in school was alphabetical. There was one other *S*, who was female, but she was *Su* and I was *Sa*, so she was way across the aisle, and I never talked to her.

The male classmates didn't know what to do with us either. Medical school was like one big fraternity network of old boys—or, rather, young boys—and the guys were all doing their thing together and we were outsiders. They may have felt threatened by us, thinking we were too smart and were competing with them to be at the top of our class. Actually two out of the seven women did end up in the top 10 percent of the class. Not me. All I wanted to do was graduate. At any rate, we were totally discounted socially.

One Friday we were in cadaver lab, and my three cadaver partners, who happened to be in the same medical fraternity, were talking about what was going on that weekend. They would talk about the girls they were going to take to the party that night, and they went on and on in front of me. It was as if I wasn't even there—invisible. And then they'd do stupid things like cutting the penis off the cadaver and tying it onto the back of a dissecting gown.

One of my cadaver partners showed some interest in me, and for that he was harassed by his fraternity brothers to the point where he wouldn't talk to me for the next three years. We never communicated after they found out. He didn't know how to deal with it. Another guy dated me and made me promise that I wouldn't tell anybody. And I actually went along with it, thinking, What am I doing this for?

But I never thought that things in medical school would ever change for women. I felt that this was simply the way it was and often wondered whether any woman would want to do this after me. It never occurred to me that someday there might be more women in school, and that they might begin asserting themselves. The same thing was true for racial integration. There was one black in our class, and he was the only person who flunked out of the medical school while I was there. And that was just the way it was.

By the third year of medical school, I figured out that 80 percent of our class was married. I did the same thing. I ended up getting married in my junior year because it was real convenient. For one thing I was depressed. I was working hard and tiring myself out, and for another my social life had gone to zilch, as I said. I had taken to staying at home without any friends, studying on Saturday night and also feeling that I wasn't attractive, that nobody was interested in me. I guess so many of us got married because in that way our social life would be taken care of. And when someone started showing a lot of interest in me I glommed right onto him. He was a physical therapy student, and he really helped me make it through school. Unfortunately, when I graduated and came out of my depression, it wasn't that much fun for him.

When the third year started and I began clerkships, I didn't see the rest of my class very much. But the clinical years were when I started to realize that I should check with the other female medical students and see what sort of problems they were having. You see, I had begun to run into sexual harassment on the wards, and I wanted to find out whether I was the only one experiencing this. On one rotation, another female student and I got into a lot of trouble because we wouldn't sleep with the resident when we were on call. We both got terrible recommendations. You know—miniskirts had just come into fashion, and we used to wear little scrub dresses which came up to here. That was the style. All I wore were clogs and my scrub dress. I'm sure that some of the residents thought we were being very seductive.

I couldn't go to the dean of the school and say, "I want you to know that this resident is. . . ." The dean would have thought I was crazy. So I checked with other women. It took me a while, but I found out that they were having the same kinds of problems, that I was not alone.

I only had one patient actually refuse to be examined by me because I was a woman. And that's not so bad. After all, a lot of women are starting to refuse examinations by men. Some of my women classmates were real uncomfortable with male patients. I knew a few who just couldn't bring themselves to do rectal exams. They all went into pediatrics.

Then there was always the problem of being confused with nurses. You can have 400 name tags and you can introduce yourself ten times as a doctor, and they'll still think you're a nurse. As a medical student I would interview a patient, take a history, do a physical, and then as I was going out the patient would say, "Nurse, could you get my bedpan, please?" I've heard of some women medical students and residents going overboard and acting more authoritarian to make sure it's clear that they're the doctor, and I've heard that sometimes the nurses don't like dealing with women residents, but all through my training I got along with nurses pretty well. I'm the kind that sits around and jokes with the staff, rather than just coming in and giving orders and leaving.

In my last year of medical school, I didn't know what field of medicine to go into, so I applied for rotating internship, since I didn't want to get pressured into anything. I moved out to San Francisco and did a rotating internship, really enjoyed it, but ended up still not being sure what I wanted to do.

There was a job opening for a GP at the university student health center, and I decided to take it. All at once I was faced with an issue that was new—the amount of money I would be making as a doctor. My husband, who was now a practicing physical therapist, wanted me to work only part-time at the health center, so that I wouldn't be making more money than he was. I went along with it—working part-time, but only because I knew that we'd be separating soon. I had begun to see that he had only been filling my needs. We got divorced soon after that.

It seems hard to be a doctor, wife, and mother at the same time. I know so few women who are doing all three of them. One friend of mine, a few years ahead of me in medical school, is married to a teacher, and she kept popping out kids during her residency in pediatrics. As far as I know, they adapted pretty well, partly because he took on a lot of the child-care responsibilities. And I'm sure people talk about him and think he's sort of strange for someone in his early forties. But if he hadn't been so flexible . . .

So many of my women friends in medicine have chosen to remain childless. I have done that. I feel I only have so much energy, and to do my job well and to be a good wife, lover, friend, whatever. If I split it further by being a mother, it would be all over. Either it would all be mediocre or one would be good and the other two would suffer. And I don't want to do that.

I worked for a year at the health center as a GP, getting very good at diagnosing and treating the big four: hepatitis, strep throat, vaginitis, and mononucleosis. I wore a white coat to make me look a little more professional, a little more asexual. I only had one bad experience tied to being a woman. It was when I was doing physicals for the football team while the usual sports physician was on vacation. Most of the players were very polite, but this one guy gave me a hard time, saying, "When do we get to examine you?"—things like that. It was obvious to me that he was on drugs; his pupils were dilated, he was spaced out, and when I confronted him with this, he denied it. I said, "Look, it is really clear to me that you are taking something." And then he said, "Promise me you won't say anything to coach?"

That year was a real turning point for me, though. For the first time I began to feel that I could do something well *because* I was a woman, not in spite of the fact. I was doing a lot of outpatient work—a lot of pelvic exams, seeing a lot of women, and getting a chance to talk with them. During my internship the patients had been almost too sick to talk, and I realized, "Hey, this is something that comes very naturally and perhaps it's something I need to pursue." By that time I was twenty-eight years old, and I don't think I'd ever had that feeling before.

At that time the women's health-care movement was taking off, and I had some friends who were involved in it who recruited me to come and work at the first free women's clinic that opened in the city. I loved the work, but I started to feel like more training would

be a good idea; Masters and Johnson had come out with their reports, and I realized there was a lot of information about sexual
counseling that I hadn't learned in college.

Through the school of public health, I arranged a residency which
fit my needs—sort of a preventive-medicine residency, with two
years of outpatient gynecology and a lot of human-sexuality training,
with family planning and genetic counseling. It was all directed
toward women's outpatient health care. It was a field I had fallen
into, which I never would have chosen in medical school, but which
was just right for me.

After I finished my M.P.H. I got an instructor's position in the
department of obstetrics and gynecology, which was real unusual,
because I hadn't done an ob-gyn residency. There were no women
ob-gyn residents at that time, and the male residents were very
skeptical about me. I'd walk in and do a family-planning clinic, or go
to the operating room and do an abortion, and they'd say, "Who is
this woman?" The thing that made them feel I was okay was that I
would take call over at the county hospital's sexual-assault center.
The ob-gyn residents didn't like coming in for rape victims, because
they didn't feel it was an educational experience. You know, the victims are hardly ever seriously hurt. Usually all you do is look for
sperm and find out whether the girl has actually been raped. So the
other residents actually got the chairman of the department to support them in not having to come in, and I agreed to take over some
of that responsibility.

I was pretty upset by this callousness, and even now I joke with
myself that my goal is to become a psychiatrist for a medical school,
so that I can take all the men who hate women and put them on a
little path that takes them toward urology—anywhere else besides
gynecology—because I'm convinced that's part of the motivation for
many of the people who go into gynecology.

Not that I can point to a lot of traumatic experiences with gynecologists in my life. My first experience with a pelvic exam was in
college when I went to the student health service, where they had a
lot of women GP's. It's a job a lot of women take because of the short
hours and the small amount of postgraduate training required. My

second experience was at the same clinic, and I had just become sexually active. The woman doctor who saw me was real pissed. She gave me the suppositories and said, "You can't have sex for three weeks"—something like that. Looking back I know that statement made no medical sense at all. Then when I was in medical school I decided I wanted to go on birth-control pills, and I went to planned parenthood because that was the only place that would give out the pill. At student health they wouldn't give out the pill unless you were married or had a note from your minister saying that you were about to marry. At planned parenthood I knew that if a person was over twenty-one she could get birth control. The first thing they did when I went in was to check my license—I was twenty-five at the time. During the examination I calmly told the examining physician that I was a third-year student. His mouth dropped, and he said nothing for the rest of the exam. I guess he thought for God's sakes, what was I doing screwing? Good girls don't do that.

During the year in which I worked at the student health center, I got involved in a nighttime family-planning clinic. There were a lot of undergraduate volunteers for the clinic, mostly women, and they were curious about going to medical school. We learned a lot from each other. I had been through medical school, and they had done things that women I grew up with wouldn't have attempted. Two of them were suing to get into the medical school. They were both over thirty, married, and they both had kids, and even though they had better academic qualifications and recommendations than most male applicants, they were not getting into medical school; it was a case of strict discrimination. That's when I became acutely aware of how stupid the medical schools were being not to accept this sort of student, and also how it was beginning to change. Both women just graduated from medical school. Jill is a medicine resident, and Karen is in ob-gyn now.

I began to find out about conditions for women inside the medical school when I was doing my year of gynecology. I set up a revised pelvic-exam course for second-year medical students. In talking to women in the second-year class, I discovered that even though there were more women than there had been in my class, there was still something missing—needs that weren't being talked about. There was the whole identity crisis of "Am I a medical student, or am I somebody's lover, or somebody's daughter?" I began to think about starting a support group for women in medicine, and now, several years later, I've finally had the time to organize one.

Ideally, the group will provide support for women to pursue their careers without the constant fear of failure or success, without having to take mediocre jobs to avoid competition with their husbands, and with the feeling that there is someone to back them up when the whole process seems too stressful. I never thought anyone was going to back me up in medical school. If I had flunked out, I felt people would have been delighted. No one would have told me, "You sue to get back in." I remember feeling that I just couldn't complain. When I was on my surgery clerkship in medical school, the surgeons had me holding retractors for eight hours at a time while they were doing some abdominal surgery. I'm not very strong, so to hold the retractor I had to lean way back—like this— and not only would I get tired, but I could never see anything. Finally I said to my professor, "I'm paying tuition to be here, and I'm not learning anything." The surgeon got real angry at me, and after that he wouldn't even let me go to the bathroom during an operation. One of my classmates used to hyperventilate so that he could pass out in the OR. That's how he would get out of the room. He'd say, "Oh God, I feel faint," and then he'd pass out. I tried it, but God, I just couldn't do it.

When I was teaching the pelvic course, a second-year medical student called me up. She had been sick and somebody had given her some Valium. The doctor who gave it to her didn't give her any instructions about how to take the Valium. By mistake—this is her story, and I feel she is reliable—she took too many, and got herself down to the emergency room and was put down as a drug overdose. For this she was kicked out of medical school. She called me, and I gave her the name of the attorney who had gotten my two friends Jill and Karen into medical school. That attorney got this student back in school within ten minutes. She just hadn't known what to do, but by calling that attorney and having someone with some power back her up, she got back in and went on to graduate without any problem. If the medical school had been allowed to kick her out on such flimsy grounds it would have been getting away with murder.

When I first came to this city, you could probably have counted on one hand the number of younger women physicians in practice here. I'm looking forward to the day when all these med-school classes graduate and everybody finishes their residencies and it is no longer such an oddity to be a woman physician. But at the same time I'm a little discouraged because even though there are so many women graduating from medical schools now, they are still going into the traditional fields. If you look at the residents at the children's hospital in town, all you see are female faces. So they're still going into pediatrics and child psychiatry. There's a need for good women adult psychiatrists, and pathology is still popular because of the flexible schedule it allows. You're seeing a few more women going into ob-gyn. In fact, three of the five ob-gyn residents accepted into the program at the university this year are women, which is a great improvement, but I still don't see that many going into surgery or the surgical subspecialties. There were two women residents in the surgical program last quarter, and they both left. I don't know if they were asked to leave or if they left by choice. If they chose to leave I couldn't blame them. The stress and the pressure is masochistic. It's got to be hard on the guys as well—it's masochistic—every other night on call. I understand that every surgery resident who started the program here got divorced by the end of his residency.

Even after the residency, I see a lot of women still choosing easier jobs like the student health services. They're not competing for the positions of power. I don't know too many women who've said, "I want to be dean of a medical school," or "I want to be chairman of a department." You don't hear of that kind of ambition. Recently I went to a meeting of a local group of women physicians. They had a cocktail party for the students, residents, and women in practice. There were about forty medical students there, about ten residents, and three practicing physicians. For the young women in practice, it seems clear that their priorities are not centered around their career. Their priorities are at home, with their family, or whatever. They aren't concerned with making an impact academically or politically—that's a lot more work.

And so, to be honest, I've been getting a little more pessimistic about changing the system with regard to women. For a long time there will be enough of the old guard around to say, "I suffered through my internship and residency, and I don't think we should make any changes." Look who's still leading everything, who's filling the positions of power.

I was back home for Thanksgiving, and I was trying to see if anything had changed at the med school. One professor of ob-gyn who literally hated women had been replaced by a very liberal guy, and they had a woman dean, though she's a psychologist and isn't paid very well. So perhaps the climate has become a little bit healthier. This kind of change seems to happen very slowly.

I visited my cousins, with whom I'm very close. They have a nice house in the suburbs. She's pregnant again and he's doing his residency in anesthesia. They have parties, and their friends come over, who are like parents I knew growing up there. The first kinds of questions I was asked had nothing to do with my career. It was usually "Are you happy?" How's your husband?" I don't get asked anymore about having kids. They know better by now.

My ten-year medical-school reunion is coming up, and I'm almost curious enough to go. Four or five years ago, I ran into one of my old classmates in the elevator, and his first question to me was "Are you still practicing medicine?" Of course, if he had run into a male classmate he would never have said that. The second question was "Do you have any kids?" And the third question was "What are you doing?" I told him I was the director of a sex clinic, just to be obnoxious, with the elevator full of people and everybody laughing.

And as long as there are Jewish mothers around, there will always be pressure on women from my background to marry a doctor, not become one!

You've Got to Show Some Concern

Donald Keith, Founder of His State's "Personal Problems of Physicians Committee"

Ellen Salzman and Matthew Steinberg talked of their personal medical journeys and the obstacles they encountered. Listening to them, I began to wonder, How common are their stories? How many physicians work too hard, lose track of relationships, come up against feelings of failure and discrimination? I reviewed the psychiatric literature on the subject of emotional distress among physicians. I expected to find some authoritative studies on the actual prevalence of suicide, alcoholism, depression, narcotics addiction, and divorce among physicians. There were virtually none.

Yet there were plenty of guesses about the extent of the problems. In 1956, America was just waking up to the problem of narcotics addiction. A physician named J. DeWitt Fox caused a stir that year when he wrote in his state's medical journal that 1 percent of the physicians in this country were narcotics addicts. With the zeal of a storefront preacher, he also advised physicians to pray daily for deliverance from the temptation of narcotics in times of stress.

Where did Fox get his figure 1 percent? He cited no studies and had personally only talked to several physician addicts. But the magic number not only stuck, it began to grow. Because it was the only estimate in the literature, it began to be quoted and before long was accepted fact. Soon the figure was 5 percent, then 10 percent.

By the beginning of the 1970s, much attention began to focus on the issue of "impaired physicians," doctors suffering from psychological distress or addiction severe enough to cripple their professional life. There were still no studies that showed how large the problem was. Many papers on the subject concluded apologetically, "Because of the reluctance of physicians to admit emotional problems in themselves and in their colleagues, the doctors who present to narcotics rehabilitation centers, alcohol detox clinics, or as suicides must be regarded as the tip of the iceberg."

I decided to talk to a doctor who was doing more than observing icebergs. I had heard that many state medical societies had set up early-detection and rehabilitation programs for "impaired physicians." The medical profession had decided to try and heal itself. I wanted to talk to one of the doctors involved in that healing.

Dr. Donald Keith was one of the first physicians in the country to both recognize the problem of impairment and start doing something about it. He divides his time between a successful suburban practice in family medicine and an active involvement in the state medical society. At his urging, the society set up a confidential "hot line" system for getting in touch with distressed physicians all over the state.

Dr. Keith's account is the story of a profession trying to take care of itself. The early efforts at dealing with impairment followed a typical medical course. This was to find the alcoholic, the narcotics-addicted, the suicidal physicians, and try to cure them.

But soon Dr. Keith saw that this was not enough. There were too many physicians with problems and not enough doctors who could spare the time to help cure them. Something more than a symptomatic approach was needed to get beyond the tip of the iceberg.

Late on a Friday afternoon, Dr. Keith's last patient having been seen, we talked in his small office in the suburbs of Seattle. In his late forties, he was a solidly built, unassuming man who spoke in a humorous but modest way. His calm, fatherly manner reminded me of a minister dedicated to steering his fold toward a better way of life.

The important thing to realize is that a medical degree does not confer mental health on an individual. Even the best of us have certain qualities that served us well in getting here. These same qualities can also allow us to break under stress. The strong, compulsive, successful physician is like an oak tree, refusing to buckle under when the wind blows. Well, great oaks don't bend, they crack.

I think of the problem of physician impairment the same way I handle other medical problems." [Dr. Keith spread his hands apart vertically in the air. As he talked he lowered his upper hand by degrees.] A person starts out at the first level, which is "no risk." The next level one descends to is "at risk," then "agent present," and on down to "signs and symptoms of impairment," and finally full "impairment."

All medical students, by the time they enter the door of medical school, have gone from "no risk" to "at risk." They're in the pressure cooker, with an extra number of demands that they didn't have before. It's devastating to get to medical school and discover that everyone else was in the top tenth of their college classes too, and now somebody has got to be at the bottom. Even the medical students who stay on top are floundering, compared to how easy they used to have it.

Oh, people may have had problems before medical school. In fact some medical students are already at level three, "agent present," when they come through the door. They may already be alcoholics.

But in terms of stress, whatever came before is nothing compared to medical school. And medical-school stress is nothing compared to residency. Things have to get a lot darker before they get any better.

After residency, physicians place the stress on themselves. The system isn't demanding it any longer, and things should get better. The physicians who get into trouble after residency are the ones who never learned how to cope with stress. They let themselves be run by their practices. For example, there's the doctor who can't say no, who's working longer hours into the evening, working on weekends. This doctor is getting an ego trip out of the way all his patients seem to love him or her, and how all the other doctors use him or her as a consultant, since "those stupid jerks couldn't get the job done by themselves." This doctor decides not to realize that the doctors are dumping off their cases because they want to go on vacation, not because this doctor is the greatest consultant in the business. Well, this kind of physician is being used by patients and colleagues. It can only go on so long. Physicians are good human beings but they have breaking points. And when they reach that point, they tend to wind up at level five, "impairment."

Nobody knows what percentage of physicians end up in that category. The figure I often repeat is that at some time in their career, 10 percent of physicians may find themselves before a medical disciplinary board. But I always repeat that with a question mark, because there just isn't any hard data. I honestly don't think that it's as high as 10 percent. The alcoholism experts estimate that 10 percent of the population in this country is alcoholic, and I'm not sure where they got their 10 percent, either. Who knows how many undiagnosed alcoholics are running around in the population?

I became interested in the problem of physician impairment in 1973, when I was both chief of staff at a hospital and a member of the board of trustees of the county medical society. I found I was having to deal with physicians whom I couldn't get a handle on. I couldn't control them. Some were just emotionally sick, some were out-and-out charlatans and rip-off artists.

At that time, there was no law that dealt with physician competency and emotional illness. If you could convict the doctor of something in court you could take their license away, but it didn't make sense to sweep the problem doctor under the rug by taking away a license to practice. It made much more sense to try and rehabilitate these people.

I proposed to the house of delegates of the state medical society that we should have some sort of statewide alerting conference to get together people who were knowledgeable about this. I naively thought that people in other parts of the country were doing a lot of things we could learn from.

We found out that the term "impairment" started in Florida in 1969 when they passed their "sick doctor" act. This law stated that when a physician acquired a license to practice, he or she gave prior consent to the state medical examining board for the board to order a medical examination whenever there was reasonable cause to believe that the physician was too impaired physically or psychologically to practice medicine safely. The board could then use that information to suspend the doctor's license.

The "sick doctor act" wasn't a closed door. The physician would have every opportunity to resume practice if he or she could prove that he or she had regained mental health.

So that was the initial law. In 1971, Texas passed one just like it, and these became the basis for the AMA's model law, which is now on the docket in thirty-six state legislatures. But even in states like Texas that have good laws, almost nothing has happened since the bills were passed.

In 1974, our state medical society held a conference on the "problem doctor" for about a hundred medical leaders from all over the state. We had people from Florida there, from Texas, from New York and New Jersey, where they were doing some things, and from the AMA, which had begun to look into the problem. We got a chance to see what had or hadn't worked in other places, and it was clear that around the country, there were still very few successful programs.

A year following that conference, the AMA presented the first rational conference on the "problem doctor"—an alerting conference. We went there and basically said, "Here's the problem, ye gods, so it is."

In Washington State we began casting around for ways to identify the physicians having problems, and if at all possible, to rehabilitate them.

Out of our statewide conference came the "Personal Problems of Physicians Committee," of which I was the chairman. We didn't use the term "problem doctor" in our title, because we had found out that impaired physicians don't like to be labeled as problems. We didn't want to offend them, to keep them away. "Disabled physician" sounded good until we thought of the guys in wheelchairs who didn't want to be lumped with the alcoholics. "Physician Support Group" came to mind, but that sounded like a firm which loans money.

We wanted the committee to be a noncoercive way of getting to doctors at an early stage, before things got too bad. The state legislature was already putting through a law similar to Florida's sick-doctor act, which was good, but it was coercive. When you look at a law that can take away a doctor's license to practice medicine, well, that law has almost the power of life and death. If you are a friend of a doctor, or a spouse or a nurse, you say, "Sure, he's got problems. But if I turn him in they'll take away his livelihood." If you're a wife, you say, "I kind of like this house, I like the style of living I've got." If you're a colleague you say, "Sure, he's a problem, but gosh, we can handle him here, and anyway, there but for the grace of God go I."

So our state Medical Disciplinary Board is very busy. They meet every two weeks, but they don't see early cases—the doctor who's been drinking heavily at a few parties. Someone like that is even hard to confront by saying, "I think you're drinking too much, Joe."

Problems were getting ignored until it was too late. That's when the Personal Problems of Physicians Committee devised the "hot line." We borrowed the concept from the state of New York, which had a great program until they changed the law. The new law said that anyone who knew of an impaired physician was required by law to report him to the state disciplinary board. That effectively destroys the noncoercive approach.

Our "hot line" is a telephone line which is in service twenty-four hours a day. When someone calls in, a recording answers, saying, "You have reached the hot-line number of the Washington State Medical Association Personal Problems of Physicians Committee." Then there's a few sentences about what the committee does, and then, "At the sound of the tone, please leave only your name, your telephone number, and the type of problem which the physician is suffering from. Do not leave the name of the physician!"

People call in from all around the state and leave their message. Usually the call comes from a hospital official or someone close to the doctor. At first we thought that doctors themselves would use the hot line, but this happens very seldom. Occasionally a doctor will call up drunk, and then when they're sober they'll regret it. And it's rare for the spouse of a doctor to call up. A few wives did, but they were in the process of divorce, and we started wondering where the complaints were really coming from.

Not even colleagues report a fellow doctor very often. Most of the calls have come from chiefs of staff of hospitals speaking for the executive committee of a hospital.

The chairman or one of the members of the Personal Problems of Physicians Committee will call the informant back and try to determine whether a problem exists. Occasionally there's no case. Say a doctor's voice was a little slurred over the phone when he gave an order to a nurse. Sure, maybe he was drunk that night, but that doesn't mean he has an ongoing problem.

Sometimes there's a case but we won't take it. A doctor may be an obvious charlatan, ripping off the public, but there's no way that we could sit down with this doctor and get him to admit that he's sick and needs help. He's going to continue to sell whatever he's selling. There's a man in town who has about a dozen little old ladies getting hydrochloric-acid drips every day. They pay a lot of money for this "IV chelation therapy," but it isn't doing them any good. This same doctor provided laetrile before it was illegal, and he draws blood and sends it through ultraviolet irradiators before reinjecting it into his patients for a price. He also likes to send his patients to little trailer courts where they can buy extremely expensive multivitamins to take care of all of their problems. He's a very interesting man, a very, very sharp charlatan, and even though he's been kicked out of the county medical society, he's still practicing and getting rich. We in the society don't have enough money to develop a case that will get the prosecutor to move on him, and we don't have enough hard evidence to drag him in front of the Medical Disciplinary Board and take his license away.

About half the time, our committee will serve in a consultant capacity. The chief of staff or the hospital administrator says, "I think we can handle it in our hospital, but we don't have much experience with this sort of thing. We need some information, some ideas." And usually they *can* handle it if we spend half an hour or so on the telephone outlining how to handle the case and what the pitfalls might be.

Finally there are the cases which warrant direct action by the committee. These are the cases where it looks like a noncoercive technique might work. So we send out a team of "confronters": two doctors who have gone through our special full-day training session on how to work with impaired physicians.

The confronters are volunteers—they donate their time. They're taught to sit back for a moment when they're offered a case and refuse to take it if they have biases. Some people are biased against alcoholics, some against sex offenders, some against drug addicts, and we want our confronters to go in with an open mind. We always send two of them out so that they outnumber the impaired physician. [Laugh] I've done some of the confronting myself.

One of the confronters calls up the physician who has been reported and says, "I'm from the Personal Problems of Physicians Committee, and Dr. So-and-So and I would like to set up a time to meet with you." They never turn us down, because the whole thing piques their curiosity. Even if they don't think they have a problem, they sure want to know what kind of goods we have on them.

During the meeting, the confronter is saying, "Look, we're trying to find out what the problem is. We've had certain facts reported to us about you; now you've got to deal with them. Either you have to tell us those facts aren't true, or you're going to have to explain to me how you came to be on the ward at that time of night swearing at the nurse or discontinuing medicines that shouldn't have been discontinued, or having a slurred voice, and why did this hospital take away your admitting privileges? I'm not shooting pool with you. I'm an official confronter. I'm coming in with a particular problem that has been brought to me, and I want to resolve it."

You keep banging away, not with rumors but with facts. Many times you can tear away the real or imagined veil of secrecy from the alcoholic or the drug abuser. The confronter is approaching the doctor from the concern of a fellow member of the state medical association, saying that "as a colleague, I think you've got a problem, and I'd like to get you some help. I can't hurt you, but I'm interested enough that I gave up part of my practice time and my family time, and it cost me some money to come over here to try to help you out."

Even if the doctor doesn't feel he or she has a problem, they are impressed by that approach. To me this is part of being a member of a profession. You've got to show some concern for other members of the profession.

Once they admit that they do have a problem, the confronter puts them in contact with a psychiatrist or an inpatient detox center, whatever, getting some type of therapeutic relationship established.

Some physicians are very willing to accept their condition. But a lot of them are wily buggers. They're intelligent, they know what their disease is, and they're difficult to confront and to treat. All alcoholics have denial, and what you're doing with the confrontation is trying to break through that denial. It may take a couple of days. You can't always do it the first time around; sometimes you have to leave your number and hope they get back to you.

If a doctor agrees to later therapy, the confronter will check back about a month after the first encounter and see whether the doctor really did what he or she said they would. "Did he really enter the detox unit?" we may ask a therapist. "*Don't* tell me whether he's doing well or poorly, just is he going at it?"

Then the confronter calls the informant and reports, "Yes, we met with him, and he's in a treatment program," or perhaps "We met with him, and he denies there is a problem."

Because we already have a coercive system for disciplinary action against physicians, the Medical Disciplinary Board, it's vital to keep the confrontation system noncoercive. If the confronter were to say, "I can't hurt you, but if you don't cooperate I'm going to turn you over to the people who can," we'd lose our early case findings. We'd be no different from the disciplinary board.

So we will never report a physician, but we do cheat a bit. We go back to the informant and say, "This physician did not feel there was a problem. If you, the informant, feel from your experience that this physician has a problem that keeps him or her from practicing medicine safely, then you should go to the Medical Disciplinary Board."

Sometimes when we report back to the informant that the physician is still denying the problem, the informant will say, "Gee, but he sure changed." So apparently we get them thinking. This isn't a permanent solution, because they tend to backslide if some therapist isn't following them. We had three or four doctors who denied problems but within a week of being confronted checked themselves into detox themselves. Maybe they wanted to do it themselves, or maybe they closed the door on the confronter and said, "What is he talking about? It's nice that he came by, but I've got no problem. I drink a little bit, but everybody drinks a bit!" Then that physician spends a few sleepless nights thinking about how much he or she is drinking, and it suddenly all falls into place, and it gets scary.

The biggest problem we encounter with the "hot line" is alcoholism. We can do something about alcoholism because everyone drinks and it's an acceptable thing to talk about.

At national conferences you hear so much about the alcoholic physician, and you start to wonder how many other problems must be out there too. Our number-two problem is narcotics addiction. Doctors have better access to narcotics than most other people. The same is true for pharmacists and nurses.

After alcohol and narcotics comes a wide range of emotional problems. Sexual offenders are one of our big problems in this category, especially among psychiatrists and anesthesiologists. I talked about this at various conferences around the country and people kept raising their eyebrows. Why was I raising this specter of sex? They didn't have any problems in their state! At one conference a man from Baltimore came up to me and said how glad he was to hear that someone else was running into sexual-offender problems. I was relieved to meet him—I didn't want to believe that my state had all the pervert doctors in the country.

Our profession has been granted a tremendous amount of latitude by society and by individual members of that society. To think that people will take their clothes off and feel reasonably comfortable, I mean really comfortable, with you! A gal can come in to her doctor and she can laugh about how she doesn't like pelvic exams—and she doesn't. But she accepts them, and the doctor can examine her and do anything he wants within reason and she feels relaxed; she trusts him, thinking, "He's going to help me." Well, there are people who are going to take advantage of that relationship!

Our committee feels that as a doctor you can do anything you want to outside of your practice, heterosexually. But when someone comes to you as a physician and you set up a romantic liaison with her, it's not the same as picking up a girl in a bar or at the church social. She and you are on unequal footing. You're coming in as the master, and she is very vulnerable, she wants help. Even if you are checking into a motel later on and thinking this is just a normal male-female affair, it isn't because she may be accepting it as part of the therapy. This is a real problem, and we're trying to crack down on it. It is a doctor's own business what he does, but not what he does with his patients.

I've been talking a lot about physicians who are men. But that doesn't mean that women in medicine don't have problems as well. At one time the women who made it through medical school did it by outmanning the men. They swore harder and told dirtier jokes than the guys did. Things are getting healthier. There's no longer the problem of breaking into the profession. The women that I run into now in medicine are competing on the basis of being a woman. When you've got 25 percent of the medical class being female, each woman can get a lot of support from the others.

But we're still seeing significant suicide among medical women, especially women residents. Women residents commit suicide three times as frequently as male residents. Perhaps the stress comes from the fact that no matter how times have changed, the woman still bears more responsibility for raising a family.

Take the woman resident who has been tired and draggy, and she calls in sick and the chief resident is swearing that "I know what she's doing. She's taking time off to get herself together, to take care of her kids." And the male residents laugh and say to each other, "Do you think we could get away with that?" But a woman does have those extra family problems. Even if she doesn't have any kids, she starts thinking, "Gee, I'm thirty, and I've got another year in my residency, and I still haven't started a family." A woman has got to be thinking about that, because at the age of thirty-five, she's an old woman obstetrically, she's got no business having babies because of the risk of birth defects. And yet here she is, thirty years old and still hasn't started a practice, still isn't making any money. Even though women tend to be more resilient and are able to bend whichever way the wind blows, they also have the extra stresses of raising a family, keeping a house, and being a doctor.

I don't have exact numbers on how many physicians the "hot line" has helped, but there have been quite a few people whom we have confronted, who have admitted a problem, gone to therapy, and several years later the lesson is still with them—they haven't gone back to alcohol or drugs. And of course there have been a lot of backsliders. Ideally, if we had enough money or enough doctors with enough time to spare, we'd monitor each doctor for years and jump them quick if they got in trouble. And ideally we would sit down with the family of the physician. Many times we find out that the spouse is depressed or alcoholic as well. We'd sit down with the family and work to reestablish their lives and give them financial advice, because by the time the doctor is in trouble they've usually ruined their practice and slid deeply into debt.

There's a lot of things that we know they need, but we can't give them everything because of the lack of time and money. I keep coming back to the fact that everybody's got to earn that living, and it's hard to ask confronters for extra time. They'll give hours, days, but we can't tie them up all the time. So I'm not at all happy with the programs we have. I like what we're doing, but we could do so much more.

It doesn't help just finding the impaired physician. You'd like to be able to prevent impairment. I'm chairman of the American Academy of Family Physicians Mental Health Committee, and one of the things we have been doing is holding "coping conferences" in various parts of the country. These conferences are for doctors at all stages of their career, helping them cope with the pressure of practice. For me, the most exciting thing about these conferences is to see so many young people—some residents, some just beginning practice. These young people aren't in trouble and they don't want to get in trouble. They've seen all the impairment out there, and they want to know how they can adjust their practices, how they can adjust their personal lives.

One basic problem, as I already said, is that the type of person accepted into medical school tends to be the same type of person as the members of the admissions committee. This successful personality is also predisposed to depression and impairment. But to get through med school and training, you need to be compulsive, you need to be able to deny yourself. So the problem starts early, and I don't see how that part of it can be changed.

But somehow, this successful person has to learn how to relax a bit, to stop being so controlling, to spend a little more time with family and friends, to allow himself or herself certain pleasures rather than putting them off.

Physicians have to learn the importance of interpersonal relationships, how to experience the love of at least one other person. Instead of doing this, doctors say, "I'll go out and buy another sports car," or "Look at all of my investments and my office buildings." They become materialistic as a substitute for affection. In the same way, they begin to abuse alcohol and drugs, saying, "Gee, I feel so wound up that I'll just take a little downer to help me sleep."

If you can love yourself and what you stand for, and if you can have real male and female friends that you can sit down with and share feelings, and if you have a spouse and a few kids who care about you, as bad as you are, that's the most important way of building support.

At present there are fewer divorces among physicians compared to the rest of the population, but there are more bad marriages. The problem gets hidden because divorce is traditionally bad for the doctor's business. If it's the husband who's the doctor, the wife tends to lose the most through divorce. Her husband is her meal ticket. Being a doctor's wife is a good social life—you get tickets to the football games, tickets to the operas, a new car. There are a lot of things that come her way, and things are fine as long as he leaves her alone and they don't fight too much. One study showed that the happiest physician marriages were the ones where the physician either spent a great deal of time at home or else was hardly ever home.

It is also terribly important to run your practice and not let your practice run you. You have to educate your patients not to call you unless there is a real need. When I first started practice, a woman called me at two A.M. to report that she was constipated. Well, that's nice. At one A.M. another woman once called me to say that her two kids had colds, "No problems, doctor, but I thought you'd want it for your records." Well, all I wanted to do was sleep. I didn't want to hear about any colds! If your patients learn to respect you as a human being, they won't bother you unless they really have to.

And you have to learn to make use of emergency rooms, of other people covering for you. You have to be willing to admit that other people can practice medicine as well as you, and that if you take a weekend off, no one is going to die under the care of your colleague.

You have to learn to say "no" to your practice, to turn it off. There are so many people in practice who can hardly wait for either retirement or the time when they can afford a partner. "If I could afford a partner," they think, "he could take part of the call." In practice everybody's got to realize that they completely control things.

I'm not a victim of my practice. All I've got to do is walk out to that girl at the reception desk and say, "Please call everyone up and book me out next week." She'll hate me [laughs], but she'll call them all up and say, "The doctor is not going to be in," and I've got a week off. I'll have no income that week, but it's my life and I can do what I want to. I can turn it off any time. I can say, "Hey, girls, I've got to go down to the medical society this afternoon; book me until twelve o'clock and then it's got to stop because I have to be downtown by one." I don't have to work through lunch, I don't have to work until seven at night because there's so many patients coming in. If I'm feeling tired I don't have to say, "Gee, it's too bad that vacation time is four months away." If I want to, I can take a three- or four-day weekend or knock out a whole week.

I have the power to do all these things. Nobody's going to sue me, nobody's going to miss me, because there's another doctor who can cover for me. You have to realize that you have that power!

PART VI

The Big Picture

"The retrospectoscope is one of the most powerful tools in medicine."

—Medical Saying

During the course of a typical year, more than three-quarters of the American population make at least one trip to the doctor. This is greater than the number who vote in a political election, go to church, or enroll in any level of schooling.

Despite medicine's continued emphasis on the individual patient and his or her particular problem, it would be impossible for some physicians not to step back and take a broader look at the immense, complex health-care process that they are a part of. That is the subject of this part: five doctors describing how they came to look at the "big picture," and, having looked, how what they saw has affected their careers and lives.

Their tone is sometimes defensive. There is a current tendency to blame America's "health-care crisis," if such a phenomenon exists, on the physicians delivering the care. "It's what I call the public paradox," an assistant secretary of HEW who was also a physician told me. "You know, the people like and trust their personal physician, and when the American Medical Association talks about medicine as the 'most respected profession,' they're dead right. But ask people how they feel about doctors as a *group* and their opinion becomes terribly negative. In the popularity polls, doctors are down around tenth or eleventh, right after longshoremen."

After so many years of comfortable insulation from public disapproval, the harsh criticism, valid or not, is making physicians react, making them assess the profession's status more carefully. They are reaping the bitter fruit of the unfulfilled promises organized medicine made in the 1950s and 1960s about how medicine, with enough public support, could effectively wipe out most diseases. It has not been that simple.

Countless books have been written on the "health-care crisis," and on the relationships of medicine, health, and society. This part supplements those many volumes of scholarly and politically astute analysis by introducing some of the physicians who have chosen to transcend the sphere of daily practice in order to try and affect events on a larger scale.

Their vantage points are often unique. They are members of a profession that unwillingly has come to reflect, even caricature, the values of the society it serves. The subtle forces of technilogical change, governmental expansion, disillusionment with the political process, and a widespread search to fill a spiritual need no longer satisfied by religion—all of these are prominent elements in the visions of these five doctors. Even the public distrust of physicians seems to be a consequence of growing consumer awareness and caution toward all professions.

Dr. Jack Carter uses his participant's knowledge about the future of computers in medicine as a model for how this country will react to computers coming to affect almost every aspect of private and public life. He reasons, with hard logic, that doctors will be among the first people to have to make great changes in work and life habits in the very near future.

Dr. William Foege, the assistant surgeon general, sees preventive medicine as the priority of the next fifty years of health care. This will have to come about through personal responsibility (such as making a decision to stop smoking) and also through effective, centralized governmental health programs such as better immunization. Dr. Foege has a right to his opinions. He directed the international effort that led to the total worldwide eradication of the smallpox virus—the first time in history that mankind has completely wiped out a disease.

Dr. Robert Hunter agrees with Foege about the need for prevention through personal responsibility. But big government makes him uneasy. He sees governmental regulation of practice in the same way Hans Roosen does, as destroying the private sanctity of the patient-doctor relationship.

Like Dr. Hunter, Dr. John Boyd is also moved by deep convictions. In the years of practice following his residency he decided that something must be terribly wrong with the American way if it was robbing so many of his patients of a decent life. Frustrated, like

Steve Seigel, in his ability to directly change things as a physician, despite his constant exposure to the problem, he has chosen to leave the country.

Dr. Benjamin Spock's life represents a more hopeful message— that change is possible. Like the other doctors who appear in this section, he became involved in larger issues through his medical work. And although his optimism has dimmed slightly since the late 1960s, he has not given up hope for the generations of young people today and in the future, upon whom he has had a lasting impact in both medical and nonmedical ways.

Computers and Medicine

JACK CARTER, PUBLIC-HEALTH PHYSICIAN,
COMPUTER PLANNER

After several hours of talking to Dr. Jack Carter, my head began to ache. Perhaps it had something to do with the relentless succession of neat, logical frames of thought he presented to me—his verbal blueprints for the future of medicine. When he talked of the current overload of information that medicine and society is staggering under, I *felt* that load. When he showed how computer technology was about to begin exploding as it never had before, I felt myself transported to a future of tactile video screens, computer consoles carried in briefcases, computer imagers watching over my shoulder.

After training in pediatrics and public health, Dr. Carter had returned to his old obsession: computers. Now he was developing a computerized records and efficiency system for a public-health hospital. And after that . . .

I had heard that Dr. Carter took notes with the lead of his mechanical pencil rolled out to an inch in length. The story went that he applied such precise and uniform pressure that the lead never broke.

The man was not far from fulfilling the myth. He opened the door of his office wearing a serious expression, as if his mind was still hard at work on a conceptual problem even as he greeted me. He was tall, thin, almost wan, and carefully dressed. Yet when he spoke he evinced an assurance and quickness, an overwhelming tide of cerebral waves. "If you want opinions about computers and medicine," he said abruptly, "you've come to the right place."

His office in the building adjoining the hospital was small but neat. A computer console stood against one wall, like a cherished piano in someone's living room. On the drafting table nearby lay several flow diagrams—algorithims for care plans, medical-record retrieval, efficient medical-history taking by paramedics.

Dr. Carter sat down in a chair next to the computer terminal, fixed his eyes on the running tape recorder, and began to emit a stream of words. Few emotions colored his tone of voice—only excitement at the possibilities for imminent progress that he saw everywhere, emphasis on the need for rational planning, and a touch of regret as he described the inadequacy of mere human minds to handle the complex tasks ahead. "Now, if I were a machine . . . ," he said.

Look—medicine is getting swamped in a sea of paper. Private doctors are beginning to charge five bucks extra just to cover the cost of processing the paperwork required by the United States government. If this trend continues, the doctor will eventually say, "Hey, I'm not willing to do all this processing. To hell with forms. I'm not going to see any patient who depends on insurance or government subsidy." And from then on, that doctor's patients will have to pay cash.

At about the same time, hospitals will wake up and say to the government, "We can't meet your information requirements. It would cost us a million dollars to put in the computer necessary to complete the reports you require. So we won't see any more medicare or medicaid patients. We won't depend on any federal subsidies; we'll give up federal funding and remove ourselves from your control."

In fact, this has already happened at some hospitals. They've also told the insurance companies, "Look, we can't afford to give you all the information you need in order to receive insurance payments from you. So we're going to take out the money and self-insure."

The point is that hospitals, insurance companies, and the government have a big investment in staying alive, and in order to maintain the status quo, they are going to have to get computerized. Computers are the only conceivable way that everyone's information requirement can be met.

Right now everyone is sitting around waiting for a system that can efficiently process all of the data; the data is waiting for the technology. There are 6.5 thousand hospitals in this country, and probably two-thirds of them have an automated billing system, since such a system pays for itself rapidly and is pretty straightforward. What hospitals are waiting for now is a similar system which can handle not just billing information, but everything—all the records. And when that happens it's going to be overwhelming, it'll sweep the country.

This won't be because the doctors want it, it'll be because the administrators and regulators want it. From their point of view computerization is a dream, a panacea. The only physicians who will really benefit will be academic researchers like myself who can put the increased amount of data to good use, who are trying to publish to stay alive. Right now I'm designing a patient-records system for this hospital. Every patient that comes to our hospital in, say, four years, will de facto be in a clinical study. Every single patient! We will not lose any data! There may not be someone who's doing the study right then, but that patient will have his data base, and he can ultimately be part of a study. Now that to me is fantastic, but it only makes a difference if it helps generate valid treatment plans.

I think that the patients will not perceive very much change at all. They'll probably be interviewed when they come in by somebody who sits by a cathode-ray tube, and the doc may actually have one in the office. But if you *really* want to automate the health-care process, the problem you're faced with is that doc who's sitting there. Let's say there's a computerized lab and a computerized pharmacy, a computerized appointment system and a computerized patient-registration system. Now you have the guts and the skeleton of an information system. The patient is associated with an ID and certain dates and a lot of numbers, which are pretty straightforward. Now you could help out the doc by giving him all this information—that's fine. But what you would really like to do is to be able to say, "Okay, doc, you're going to generate all this history and physical exam and your plans. What we want is to be able to take that text you're creating and turn it into numerical codes, and store them as if they were lab data."

There are a lot of ways to do this. The doc can do it by filling out an encounter form, where he checks off different boxes on a sheet, and each box represents a sign or symptom and has an assigned code, and then the sheet is put right into the computer; fine. The problem with it is that a lot of docs don't like to be crammed into little boxes. But the encounter forms will do about 90 percent of the job for about 10 percent of the cost, and this kind of low technology will be the solution for handling common problems which are straightforward. The problem comes in that final 10 percent, the complicated patient or the weird problem. I think you'll find when you get out in practice that 90 percent of what you see is the same old bullshit. Every doc, every doc who's in practice has his bread-and-butter patient who has a straightforward problem that the doc understands well, and who makes money for him because he sees him rapidly. Every doc also has complicated patients that are interesting that cost him money. All the computers will do is help him take care of those complicated patients. Well, how to do that is indeed a big problem.

There's a guy in Vermont named Larry Weed who's come real close. He uses a computer terminal that has sensitive areas on a screen which you touch to choose which information you want accessed. It's called making selections from a menu. Now say a doctor wants to do a physical exam. The first menu of the entire system asks what do you want to do: a history, or physical exam, or problem list. The guy touches the screen and says, "I want to do a physical exam," and boom, the screen fills up and says "Okay, you're doing a physical exam, what part do you want to start with—head, eyes, ears, nose? All right, head, what do you want to say about the head?" The computer uses these frames that are flashed up very rapidly to allow a person to go right through a physical exam.

Weed's menus are very nicely done. He has 40,000 different frames, okay? It really is incredible. His whole trip is that you could force people to follow a logical train of thought by using this system, because you're presenting them with the links in a chain, and if they skip something they get stuck. So by going through this, they learn what is expected; they learn to do a complete history, a complete physical exam, and they're forced to follow patterns of logical thought that are set up by specialists in the field, people who know all about various problems. It will be very useful for training docs, because a person can say, "I'm right here in my physical exam, but I don't know how to do this," or "I forgot." And the computer says, "Well, here's how to do it," or "Here's an article on the subject." It will also be very useful for diagnostic problems and esoteric diseases. Also, doctors don't spend very much of their time on those things. They are trained by the time they get out, and the vast majority of their practice is not rare, it's quite understandable. When you get out there and you see five patients of a certain type, you know the stuff.

Weed has worked out a very nice principle, but there are areas in which it becomes very cumbersome. For one, it's extremely high technology, requiring very specialized and expensive electronic equipment. What's more, you may have to run through 300 frames to do a physical exam, or 300 frames to do a history. Even at high data rates, even with very slick technology, the providers who use it will get real tired of whipping through frames.

What you need is a hybrid system that will use menus for complicated problems or for training people, and a more free-form technique which will allow the provider to enter data as computer text. The computer then cross-references the input line and tries to figure out what the hell the doctor is trying to say. This is what I'm working on now.

I've defined any contact point between a patient and the medical-care system as a medical event, and I feel that if you have eighteen different variables you can define the context of any conceivable medical event. Take a nosebleed, for example. Two dimensions of that would be the part of the body affected and the function that's affected. In other words, the nose, and bleeding. Now, some other dimensions of that event would be the time at which it started, the time that it's being seen now, the person who's seeing it now, the periodicity of the symptom, does it come and go, the severity of the symptom on an arbitrary scale from one to four plus, and so on. If you think about it for a while, you'll see that most things in medicine have these dimensions; it's quite systematic. Even with a lab test you can say it had an onset when it was done, a severity which is its value compared to the normal. You can use normalized numerical values that are standard deviations from the average for that age group, and so on. Then you can use an n-dimensional rank to store a long number that completely defines a medical event, and that number takes up seventy to eighty bits in the machine, or something like that, so in a very compact manner you can completely define any intersection of a patient and the medical-care system.

Let's say [he sits down at the computer console] that I am in the clinic and I see a child with epistaxis—nosebleed. I type in . . . epistaxis . . . that's two dimensions right there, then, onset, oh, three days ago . . . three . . . D . . . A . . . , then the fourth dimension, which I can't conceptualize, is severity . . . three plus . . . then periodicity . . . P blank C . . . constant, and blah, blah, blah. If I knew the eighteen dimensions, if I were a machine and had them in my head, I could in theory run through them each time without leaving any out. In practice, the computer can prompt the doctor and say, "Hey, you forgot to say anything about onset." So it's possible that certain providers may be able to enter this kind of data at a keyboard just as if they were taking notes on a piece of paper. The computer would interpret that and spit it out in the English language.

The hybrid system is going to end up being the most viable because providers are different; some are sophisticated, some aren't, some just want to throw some shit in there and not care about it, some want to be very complete, and so on. This hybrid gathering system will ultimately eliminate the untrained lower clerical personnel in the interface between the doctor and the machine. There's something like a 10 percent error rate when secretaries sit down and type things into the computer, because they don't know anything about medicine. I want to eliminate that kind of bad data.

However, another advantage of computer implementation is that it allows a new group of providers to function in a safe manner. You can validate treatment protocols and have low or moderately trained people doing specific tasks that are monitored by the computer to keep track of how well they do in terms of adherence to the algorithm. Who gains from that? Well, the patient gains, because the system would be using people that earn a third of what a doctor earns, and they would be gathering about ten times as much data and spending about the same time with each patient. Of course, it's a tradeoff. The patient loses the support that comes from personal contact with a physician, you know: "I talked with a physician, he said my kid was okay." But I have data which shows that paramedics do as good a job as docs on any criterion that you can measure. They do the same or better.

The hospital administrator gains from this because it costs him less to deliver care, the regulatory agencies gain because their net expenditures for health in the country are reduced, and the physician loses out because his job is being taken away. I just can't stress this enough. When you look at the ultimate impact of computers on medicine, you have to look at it on a group-by-group basis. There's the government, there's hospitals, there's patients, and there's health-care providers of all kinds. The ones who stand to lose from computerization are the docs—everybody else gains. Doctors have the most to lose since their privacy will be invaded; in fact, it will disappear. They will be monitored very closely, and all they will gain is this amorphous, intangible, undocumented, purported benefit to the patient coming from a greater data base. The idea is that doctors will be able to provide better care.

You know, no other profession is going to be watched as closely as physicians will be. The peer-review system as it currently stands is nonsense, I mean it's just trivial. They sample 1 percent of charts and look them over and say, "Ah, this looks okay, you know, blah, blah." Well, imagine when every chart can be monitored, when peer-review criteria are enforced, when you put something in the computer and it bounces back at you the next morning on your desk. I don't think anybody has prepared for the incredible professional fight that there is going to be over that. I think that docs are justifiably angered by the assumption that they practice lousy medicine until proven otherwise. Don't forget that nobody outside of medicine realizes that doctors aren't perfect, and that in fact any time you do a test the test has a finite chance of being wrong, and any time you make a decision there is a finite chance that you're wrong. We doctors deal with a probabilistic view of the world, and we are going to be wrong, dammit. If private juries sit out there and assess quarter-of-a-million-dollar damages for the finite number of mistakes that occur, medicine's going to go out of business. There has to be not only a change in peer review, but at some point the legal system has to take a much more sophisticated point of view toward malpractice; otherwise this whole thing is gonna go bananas. There isn't a doctor in practice today who hasn't actively hurt a patient by virtue of a mistake.

This whole issue has not been faced, and the computer is going to bring it up and shove it in people's faces. The profession is I think justifiably alarmed, because there's no evidence so far that anybody really is doing anything about it that is rational, that anybody really cares. Doctors look at the fact that they're gonna have a little electronic gremlin sitting on their shoulder saying, "Hey, you know you gave that penicillin, and the dose is a little bit too high." They will go, "Oh my god, some jury could look at that, and I could get my ass sued." And so what's going to happen is they're just gonna go into this shell, and either not do things, or they'll do everything four times to be sure that they're all covered. We physicians have fostered this aura of being perfect, and now it's coming back at us.

So is there anything in it for doctors? Well, most docs will tell you that they would spend more time with their patients if they could. Not all of them feel this way, but I think that's a pretty general feeling especially among younger physicians. I'm hoping that the computer would allow that. It takes away a lot of the bullshit and makes some time for other things. Maybe it's fair to say that the patient gains and the physician breaks even on the deal.

It all depends on what you want from life as a physician. The computer will cut down the need for docs. It will hopefully enrich their practices because it will take away a lot of bullshit care. Ten years from now, as a pediatrician I could put myself in a clinical setting where I didn't have to see every runny-nose kid that came into my office. On the other hand, a lot of guys stay alive doing that. The computer will mean this country will need fewer specialists, since all docs will be specialists, but it will make their lives better. If we have fewer physicians twenty years from now their lives would be a hell of a lot more interesting and useful to society.

Curing the World

WILLIAM FOEGE, ASSISTANT SURGEON
GENERAL, DIRECTOR OF CDC

William Foege was back at his medical school to receive its first Distinguished Alumnus award. The morning before the honorary luncheon, he sat surrounded by a few local newspaper reporters. His clean-cut, all-American good looks jarred with the exotic flavor of his stories, the place names like Senegal, Somalia, Dahomey, India. Yet woven into the accounts was a steady thread of medical facts, agricultural probabilities, economic forecasts: the verbal toolbox of a physician deeply involved in public health.

As director of the CDC program that contributed to the international effort to eradicate smallpox from the world, Dr. Foege developed a systematic, focused attack plan. Concentrating resources to areas of outbreak, he had guards stationed for six weeks outside the quarantined house of a victim, while a thorough sweep within a ten-mile radius for other cases was performed, and all local villagers received vaccinations. Because the smallpox virus requires a human host, this method had immediate results. The eradication effort spread across twenty countries, employing millions of health workers and volunteers. In one week of operations in India, 11,000 cases were discovered. And slowly, one country at a time, smallpox began to lose its grip. The last natural case appeared in October of 1977. "And now," said Foege with a self-assured tone, "the job is finished. When the World Health Organization inspection team declares Somalia smallpox free this fall, it will be the first disease in recorded history to completely disappear."

Now Foege was both assistant surgeon general for the United States and director of the Center for Disease Control in Atlanta, Georgia. It was the CDC whose workers unraveled the mystery of legionnaire's disease, the strange pneumonia that caused more than twenty deaths following an American Legion convention in Philadelphia in the summer of 1976. Using blood samples stored at the CDC, investigators tied legionnaire's disease to five other unexplained outbreaks since 1947. From the lung tissue of a Philadelphia victim, they finally isolated a new species of pathogenic bacteria, *Legionella pneumophila*. Foege smiled at the recollection. "I believe that I've experienced directly the thrills of a Pasteur or a Koch. It proves that medicine is dynamic and understandable. We've seen decades of common sense at its best. We keep climbing on the handholds and footholds which are challenges successfully met. At present, of all the infectious diseases only influenza is on the list of top ten killers in this country."

The reporters drew their chairs closer, pencils poised. Were there any more miracles in the offing? Foege grew instantly more reserved, pushing away the air in front of him with large hands. Yes, he conceded, there was some cause for optimism with the new flu vaccines, and the school-entrance requirement for measles vaccine had brought the incidence down to 10 percent of the usual rate. But more miracles? He shook his head. "I'm a scientist, not a wizard."

The reporters excused themselves, appearing disappointed. Dr. Foege pushed back his chair and unfolded his long legs. "That feels a lot better," he sighed. "I get cramped in these chairs." He smiled to himself. "When I was on the smallpox project, I asked an African village chief to send a message over the talking drums to have as many people as possible come to the village for vaccinations. He agreed, and within an hour the square was packed solid with people. I turned to the chief and asked, 'How did you get them to come so fast?' 'It was simple,' he replied, 'I told them to come see the tallest man in the world!'

"You know, one thing I've decided while I've been back here at my old medical school is that med school prepared me for my career as an administrator, even though there were never any courses in management and I never thought I was acquiring those skills. But coordinating a patient's care taught me all sorts of subtle lessons about working with a team of people to solve a medical problem. All that happened in my career was that the teams got bigger and bigger." He chuckled.

But you know, I expected to be a general practitioner—that's what I was aiming for. Then as I went through medical school, I made some very conscious, objective decisions about what field I should go into. I picked public health, because it seemed like the right thing to do, even though I wasn't sure I was interested in it.

If you look at the increase in longevity in this country—twenty-six years added to the life span since the turn of the century—it looks dramatic, and you assume that yes, American medicine is great. People quote these figures all the time.

But at my age, I can only expect about four and a half more years of life than my grandfather could have. The big change in longevity comes from the fact that babies and infants no longer die at the same rate they did in 1900. Why aren't they dying? It comes down to five or six very distinct things that have happened. We now have protected water supplies. We now have sanitation systems. We now have food laws that make it likely that the food you give to your children won't have typhoid or salmonella in it. We have better nutrition—you can't over-estimate the role of malnutrition in disease. The leading cause of death in West Africa is measles, and the primary reason is not just the measles virus, it is malnutrition *plus* the measles virus.

And finally you add immunizations to that list of factors. This is the only contribution that American medicine has made to the reduced infant mortality, and heck, you don't need doctors to give immunizations. One health planner has said that if we were to lose all hospital beds overnight in this country, it wouldn't have the same impact on the nation's health as losing one of the preventive measures I just listed.

So even though it wasn't my first love, I decided to go into preventive medicine. Secondly, I decided to go into preventive medicine as it affects the third world, since that's the place where a unit of resource, whether it's time or money, can do the most. Once I got involved in preventive medicine, it turned out happily that I became so absorbed that after fifteen years I sat down and objectively tried to look at my career and decided I seriously could not think of something I would have preferred doing in the last fifteen years. So that turns out to be an added benefit, but I didn't go into it because I thought I was going to get a lot of personal pleasure; I went into it because it looked like a rational, scientific, objective decision.

One of the questions we should ask as individuals and as a professional group is what is the purpose of medicine? It comes down, I think, to two things, to prevent what can be prevented and to deal with what can't be prevented.

American medicine has been superb in dealing with what can't be prevented, and it's hard to put a price tag on the morbidity and mortality that's been alleviated. There's so much that you just can't prevent, but we have to keep asking ourselves what can we provide with fewer resources? What are the priorities? How do we get traditional individual medical ethics broadened to look at societal medical ethics? Everything you'll be taught in medical school will be at a bedside, where you are taught that you must do the most you can for this person. If you start looking at societal ethics, you'll see that you're paying a price somewhere else. After all, one heart transplant can probably be equated with 10,000 person-years of life if you used that money for measles vaccine in West Africa.

American medicine is a luxury that can't be afforded in most countries until they develop their basic prevention procedures. At one time we thought that we could bring the rest of the world to our standard, but now I think if there is to be any equity in the world it will involve a decrease in our own standard, and this includes medicine. At the luncheon today I'm going to tell some little stories on medicine and history. One of them will be looking ahead 100 years and asking what will historians think about the way we made choices? when we got so upset about saccharin but not about cigarettes? when we were able to get rid of measles in this country but didn't do it in Africa? Will we look back 100 years from now and say,

"you know, that was no different from the mentality of slavery?"
We've still got the haves and have nots, and we still do not understand that society eventually benefits by having some equity.

Another approach is to look forward and ask where we will see our
gains in the next fifty years. If you take the ten leading causes of
death now, they come down by and large to four generic causes; cigarettes, alcohol abuse, improper diet, and accidents. Then suddenly
you realize that with all four of these we're not waiting for new
research breakthroughs—we already know how to prevent them. A
thousand people die each day in this country because of cigarettes.
So the next fifty years will still be prevention, but where I see a
change is in the fact that prevention in the past has been largely
social manipulation. Prevention in the future will be a combination
of social manipulation and the acceptance of personal responsibility.

When I say social manipulation I mean doing things about the environment of the individual patient—sanitation, food safety, and so
forth. Now there is no way to do this without a strong central government. There is no way that you can draw up priorities for the
country, then implement them by giving tax breaks if people do the
right thing. If you want to get labels put on food telling the cholesterol content, there's no market incentive for that unless you have a
strong central government saying that's what should be done. And
when it comes to personal responsibility, you need a national health
insurance of some kind to ensure that poor people have the same
access to preventive-care services. I don't see any way to overcome
the inequities for the disenfranchised unless someone is ensuring
that they will be able to come for care—and this doesn't happen in
the marketplace. You don't see the marketplace taking care of poor
people in the grocery area by saying, "We'll make food cheaper for
poor people—you just come in and tell me whether you're rich or
poor and I'll adjust the price." That doesn't happen. If you ensure
that poor people have insurance and access to the system, then if
they don't want to use it that's their personal choice. But now they
can't make a personal choice.

It's amazing how ten and twenty years later we always look at
these things and wonder why people didn't understand. I think that

Will Durant is right. We are evolving upward, not up and down, up and down; we are evolving upward and we continuously get insights that we didn't have a decade ago. At some point we will see this for health in this country, and at some later point we will understand it on a global basis.

Of course, there's still a need to take care of the things that couldn't be prevented or weren't prevented. You can't abandon someone at age fifty because their life-style brought them to the brink of disaster. But we have to make personal decisions on where we want to be in this overall theme, and at this point I get my pleasures and joys from being able to see the measles curve go down. I don't have any trouble translating that to real people in my mind. Public health is simply personal health multiplied by X number. That doesn't mean I'm immune from the seductions of clinical medicine, because they're there and I feel them. All I had to do some years ago was go back to Africa, where I had been practicing, and to see the gratitude of people whom I had treated, to realize that the daily feedback really is seductive.

Working in Africa, where health problems are so widespread, there was always the feeling of being overwhelmed. Many people I have seen overseas reacted by working harder than you've ever seen people work—literally all day long. But these people are always dealing with the numerator—the sick people who come to them. The only way I could maintain my mental health was to say, "I'm going to look at the denominator; I'm going to try and figure out what are the biggest problems. Where can I make a contribution that would be lasting? I'll draw up some priorities and go to work!" I still ended up working hard, but it wasn't the same sort of always being overwhelmed and not seeing the bigger picture.

With the smallpox project, I was convinced of the possibility of eradication before I even knew I was going to be involved. In 1967 it became clear to me—I knew it was going to happen. My celebration was back when I first knew it was possible. Many people felt like celebrating when the last case occurred in a particular country, but I always had a different feeling. Had I celebrated when it actually happened, that could have indicated I had some doubts.

I tend to see diseases in a very simplistic way. Sure, we were fooled many times during the smallpox program and the legionnaire's-disease investigation, but I never believed in something that was irrational. It wasn't spontaneous generation. There was an explanation, though we didn't always find it. Sometimes when we were baffled by a real mystery something would appear that explained it, and then we could say, Well, I bet that's what happened before, and we missed it." There's something similar going on now. Can we break measles transmission in this country? A lot of people believe that it's impossible, or that it's going to be an awfully difficult job. But to me, it's just logically possible. If you can get enough children who aren't susceptible, you can't have measles transmission.

There's no question that there is cause and effect in this universe. You notice that the direction of our knowledge is always to solve mysteries. We didn't understand hepatitis B two years ago. And now, all of a sudden a light bulb goes on, and of course there's a third strain here. We've been confusing B and non-B strains. We keep getting more information, and that leads to the light bulb. It doesn't go the other way around. It's not often that more information obscures something that was clear before. This leads me to believe that there is a rational basis for things that happen, and it's simply a question of eliciting the right information. You know Einstein had that feeling in physics, and that's what kept him going on that general field theory—that God doesn't play dice with the universe. I believe the same thing, but that it's a challenge to find out what those causes are. I don't believe in witchcraft.

The AMA

ROBERT HUNTER, AMA PRESIDENT-ELECT

In 1847, 250 physicians met in Philadelphia to form the American Medical Association. Their hope was to raise allopathic medicine far above the host of competing healing philosophies: naturopathy, homeopathy, osteopathy, and chiropractic. Great discrepancies in training and almost no formal licensing had left American doctors with a social, economic, and professional standing far below that of their European counterparts. "Therapeutic nihilism" was on the rise, as the public wondered whether physicians were doing more harm than good.

The long path from 1847 to the present was marked by such events as the rise of Flexnerian medical schools, increasingly strict licensing requirements, the postwar boom of technological medicine, and the battles over medicare and medicaid during the 1960s.

"The AMA . . . Working for You," reads the shiny membership brochure mailed to physicians and medical students around the country. "The standard bearer of excellence . . . since its inception, the AMA has provided the leadership which has led to the excellence of medical education and the high quality of medical care in this country."

Whatever its contribution to history, the AMA receives $250 in yearly dues from almost half the physicians in the United States. It remains the strongest voice of organized medicine and one of the most powerful lobbies on Capitol Hill.

The Hunter Clinic is a drab, one-story building off the main street of Sedro Wooley, Washington. This small farming community seems an unlikely place for one of the most powerful figures in organized medicine to have an office, but Robert Hunter smiled at the suggestion. "Don't forget," he said with a trace of humor in his deep voice, "Sedro Wooley is no smaller than Plains, Georgia."

The spring-morning sun shone through the window of his modest office. He was home from one of his frequent trips. "I just testified before the Congress. They wanted to know what the AMA's stand was on the public-health effects of smoking. As the chairman of the board, I reaffirmed the AMA's strong feelings about the hazards of cigarette smoking. Then I went on a fact-finding trip to the Philippines, examining their health-care system. I got off the plane yesterday and resected a colon in the afternoon."

He spoke in the careful, sonorous tones characteristic of a public figure. Among AMA regulars, his massive build and firm, blocklike features had earned him the nickname "the Gorilla." But Dr. Hunter was not one to beat his chest or rage openly. His power was an unspoken aura, a reserved yet unyielding force.

He adjusted his steel-rimmed glasses, then rested huge hands on the glass-topped desk, fingers entwined. "I'm grateful to my brother for filling in for my deficiencies here, since I am away more than two-thirds of the time. Our practice is truly a family tradition. My father came to this town as a physician fifty years ago, and some of his patients are now my patients. I feel there is a great mutual benefit in this kind of long-term, personal relationship. The townspeople come from good solid stock and have medical problems that are fairly straightforward; heart disease, some cancer, some diabetes. There is little acute poverty, and almost no medicaid patients, but many of the older patients receive medicare. Yes, I still make house calls when it is imperative, and I run my general surgical practice with the utmost regard for my patients. Having a practice here keeps my hat size from getting too big, and no patient of mine has to sit more than fifteen minutes in my waiting room!"

On the wall of his office, plaques of appreciation from local community groups were interspersed with photographs of Robert Hunter shaking the hands of presidents, Robert Hunter making speeches.

He was silent for a moment, thinking over his original decision to become a doctor. Then he told his story, steadily, calmly.

My father was in the military corps at the time I was born, and until I was ready to finish high school I wanted to be a regular military officer myself. But suddenly the urge hit me that I wanted to go to medical school, and I've never looked backwards or regretted the decision. I finished my premedical education at the age of nineteen, went through medical school when I was twenty-three, which gave me a leg up on others and several years of practice experience in addition to what most doctors my age have.

I suppose what got me involved in politics was the weariness of the physicians who were left home during World War II. They had kept medical associations, societies, and organizations alive in the absence of probably most of the younger physicians who were in the military. I can remember when I first came back home and my father took me to my first county-society meeting. There were four or five other young doctors who had arrived almost simultaneously, and the older men were very willing to hand over the organizational obligations. Being young Turks, we were glad to take hold of it. This meant that very early on we were elected to office within the county society. Finding that of interest, I went on to involvement in the state medical association, from there to the national picture, and now I've served in really every chair of the county, state, and national organization except one, and that may become a reality come July, when I'm a candidate for president-elect of the American Medical Association.

My only prior conception about all of this was that within a few years I was either going to go up or go out. Twenty-five years ago, I said I would spend ten years at the level I was at, and then either be elected to a higher level or move over and let somebody else have a run at it. That has proved out, and my eight-year service on the board of trustees of the AMA has been the longest time I've spent at any one level. The last two have been marked by being chairman of the board, and that job has much more in the way of responsibilities and time demands.

One of the things that you will come to realize is that our profession makes up a highly selective population that is academically superior, theoretically morally superior, placed in a position of trust and confidence by our patients; but it is still a profession composed of individuals, each one thinking that his opinion is meritorious and should be the opinion of the whole profession. It's hard to give up any of those individual rights and individual judgments in favor of the judgment of the profession altogether. Now, this leads to decisions between specialists and general practitioners; it leads to turf conflicts within the specialties that sometimes are very difficult to overcome. Most people should realize that if you are in agreement 90 percent of the time, the 10 percent disagreement is no reason to pick up your marbles and go home. The 90 percent is a good reason to stay in a unified effort.

Often it isn't so much a matter of theory as it is attitudes. Of course, during the sixties I saw this tremendous thrust toward anti-establishment and rebellion that affected medical schools as well as other areas of medicine. I deplored that because I feel that I am part of the establishment, and any rebellion against the establishment was a rebellion against me and what I represented. In the last few years I've seen a very definite swing back—you have neither mustache nor beard, you're wearing a white shirt and a necktie. And I'm sure that's commonplace amongst your classmates, but ten years ago, if they weren't in blue jeans and an afro and bearded and insolent, they didn't seem to belong.

Was I that way when I started out? Not at all, not at all. I worked within the establishment. And I think that this is the lesson that the young physicians have learned now. After all, the president of the Los Angeles County Medical Association, over 8,000 members, is about thirty years old. He has learned to work within the establishment. And you should be interested to know that the fastest-rising component of membership in the American Medical Association in the last five years has been medical students.

I would say that the primary consideration of the organization now is the cost of health care. Of course, every element in society has contributed to the escalation of cost, not the least of which is government itself, but also industry, labor, the insurance industry, and the providers of health care. Physicians are partly responsible, hospitals are partly responsible. The trend in America has been to provide the best available care to as many of our citizens as we can. This is the second-largest industry in the country, exceeded only by agriculture as far as dollars involved or number of people working within the industry. There's no way that it can be inexpensive. But Secretary Califano of HEW says simply that hospitals are an obese industry and that dollars should be wiped off the top because they can exist on less. Well, that isn't the answer. Hospital expenditures are 70 percent for labor, and who's to say that the people working in a hospital are making too much money? Perhaps greater efficiency, greater productivity can be achieved, but you know a wholesale slash of people and their income is not the answer to rising hospital costs.

A current trend is that we as physicians are asking the citizens of this country to assume personal responsibility for their own health, the preventive measures of self-help and . . . oh . . . responsibility for weight, smoking, auto accidents, diet, et cetera. Particularly the young people want to know why, they want to know what, they want to know what options are available, and I can't argue with this; I think it's simply expanding the relationship between doctor and patient. But when consumerism is expressed through an outside agency, such as Ralph Nader or Sidney Wolfe, I object strongly to it. Sidney Wolfe, head of Nader's Health Research Group, has never taken care of a private patient in his life. He has no reason to comment on the practice of medicine, because he's not a part of it. And there's an old saying: If you haven't bought a ticket, don't complain about the railroad.

A lot of people don't understand the doctor's position, and this is particularly true of Secretary Califano, who is in a never-never land, and congressmen, who whenever they see a problem, they throw a law at it. Secretary Califano, I think, can be classified as a hip shooter, and if he sees a problem he throws an idea at it. Too often it's his own idea, and being a practicing attorney, his knowledge is not sophisticated or broad enough to know how complex some of the problems he's trying to answer are, and how interwoven the solutions have to be.

The threat that doctors always feel is in the background is that dark cloud of governmental interference, the threat of a governmentally controlled profession. There's no question about it, after World War II we had four regulatory agencies in the federal government. We now have seventy-eight. And that isn't just a regulation in the medical profession, it's a regulation of every facet of our lives. It affects business, labor; it results in increasing taxes; it results in an ever expanding governmental employment; it results in more paper coming out of Washington and more paper that has to flow back to Washington. It's a matter of setting up parameters of behavior that stifle individual freedoms and individual responsibilities.

Within the past year, I've had the opportunity to visit Red China, Japan, Australia, England twice, South Africa, and Brazil, and I found that where there is governmental intervention in the medical profession and increasing government regulation, the tendency is always to reduce the scope of benefits and the quality of service for everyone to the lowest level rather than raising the lowest level to that of the highest quality, high performance, high access. In England their facilities are deplorable; the people are months waiting for services. In Canada, where there is an ever increasing involvement of the federal government and the provincial government, it is leading to the closure of medical schools, the closure of hospitals, and in truth cannot help affecting the quality and access to services.

In July of that year, the AMA House of Delegates convened at the plush Chicago Marriott Hotel, which was partly owned by the organization. At seven o'clock in the morning of the opening session, Dr. Hunter sat at a breakfast meeting with his state's delegation. "I have the honor," he intoned, "of running without opposition for the office of president-elect. It's a good, warm, comfortable, satisfying feeling."

Throughout the week he moved serenely above the infighting and political haggling over AMA policy. The 700 delegates unanimously opposed national health insurance, they divided over whether to label chiropractic an "unscientific cult," and they moved to increase membership among women and medical students. "Our polls show that 64 percent of the general public places fair or great trust in the AMA to find solutions to our health-care problems," stated the outgoing president. "Why aren't an equal percentage of physicians supporting us? We need 20,000 new members each year just to keep up with inflation."

Leaving the Country

John Boyd, Family Practitioner

John Boyd was filling in for vacationing doctors around the city, earning enough money to get by while he planned his trip to Mozambique. The newly established Socialist government was badly in need of medical advisers.

But the fact that Dr. Boyd was American made the Mozambiqueans wary. They wanted to be sure that he was not an informant for the CIA. They wanted to be sure that he was married to his female companion.

Over the past months, Dr. Boyd had passed their scrutiny, won their official trust. He hadn't planned to get married so soon, but this move to Mozambique was something he was committed to.

Two weeks before his departure, Dr. Boyd took time off from his preparations to discuss with me his reasons for going. They seemed to spring from a deep need to *live* according to his principles, his convictions. Almost wearily, he acknowledged that this had not been possible as a physician in this country. His medical career had given him a political awareness but no tools with which to effect change.

We sat outside on a grassy hillside that was beginning to warm to the spring sun. He was softspoken and scholarly in his manner, but his arms were thick from exercise. There was a constant anger simmering under his words, and as he moved his hands in the air, I could see that his knuckles were scarred.

"From punching walls during medical school," he had explained. Taking a sip of coffee, he began to share his story.

I think people's experiences and particularly struggles are what politicize people, and not just isolated events. My last year at Harvard was when I got my first dose of marxism. It was a pretty heavy time, you know, when the cops busted the students who were occupying the administration building. I was interested in the occupation, and hanging around the administration building, but I wasn't interested enough to spend all night there and wait till the cops came. I guess one way of figuring out one's political perspective is to find whether you're willing to stay up all night.

I went to medical school because I would have been drafted. My father's a doctor, and I saw what he did, and it didn't seem like that big of a deal, but I was always gonna be a doctor, and here the war was gonna knock me in, so I decided that well, I might as well.

My school was in Chicago, and I started working for the Black Panthers there. Maybe ten people in my class did that, so it wasn't any big deal, but we went out and did home surveys and started realizing that there was some real poverty, some real real shit going on, not just poverty but alienation. The blacks sure were in the pits as far as our society was concerned, though of course they weren't as bad off as people in India. Just then, Cambodia happened, and I got politically involved within the med school and was surprised at how few of the people around me were responding in the same way. That was my first dose of peer struggles, trying to get people together to make a statement and finding that other people's reasons for becoming doctors were separate from any awareness of social problems.

It started affecting me, and when I got into clinics it got worse because I started realizing that medicine was disconnected from what seemed to be going on. You were helping certain people with certain diseases, but most of the people who had those diseases had them for other reasons. You don't see pneumococcal pneumonia very often except in alcoholics. You don't see subacute bacterial endocarditis very often. It's the classic disease for medical students to learn. You get all these physical findings. Everybody wants to see it. Well, you know, it happens in drug addicts—they're the people who get it. I began to realize that medicine is simply a pit stop where people who are having trouble with society can drop out for a while by getting sick.

Being a doctor is like being a cop. Doctors are social policemen, in a way; they are judges of society, judges of humanity. They're very strongly involved in identifying people who are deviant in society and in saying that there is a particular reason for their deviance. It comes out of a framework of illness. You become a social policeman by saying to many, many people whose primary cause of illness is social, "No, your primary cause of illness is individual." This forces the patient to say, "Yeah, there's something wrong with me, and I've got to deal with it." Medicine runs on the same principle as Alcoholics Anonymous. That "this is a disease, and it's your personal responsibility to take care of things." Even holistic health tends to operate on these lines. It says, "You know we've got a bad society, but the problem is you have got to deal with how you fit in society." It's an easy trap to fall into, because in medical school I was taught that I was better than most people at perceiving people's needs— that's the doctor's specialty. Well, unfortunately that's wrong, because actually my expertise lies in a few specific pieces of medical information and skills. I mean, you can't say that all of medical knowledge is bullshit, but at the same time it's limited, totally limited within the context and the framework of the society you're dealing with.

In practice I saw a lot of working-class people who had a very difficult time in their jobs. They really didn't have very much self-esteem at all, and they got sick right after they changed their shifts. There was a study done by HEW called *Work in America*, and it concluded that the most important prerequisites for health were job satisfaction and a general sense of happiness. Now, these are hard to put your foot on. You can't say to a patient, "You've got to be more satisfied at work," you can't say, "Well, you've got to unionize." I'm frustrated because in this country I don't have any obvious avenues to go, trying to change things as a doctor.

I'm also tired of the temptation to sell out. That's touching on one of my major fears: the urge to be comfortable. When I got out of my residency I worked in a clinic where I made $3,200 a month just for showing up for work—it was incredible: I live simply. My car is an old one that I bought six years ago for $500, and I live in a house where my total bill for rent, utilities, and food comes to $200. I started thinking, wow, it's really fun to watch my bank account grow—that's a lot of money to be salting away.

Once during the holiday season I worked a day covering for a friend in an emergency room. For one day's work—I guess he was paying me double time—I made $1,000. So I can understand my classmates settling into fairly comfortable practices and not becoming too political. I get judgmental sometimes, but I can understand wanting to be comfortable. When I'm old I will want some security, I won't want to be working hard to stay alive. But right now, I want to stay aware of what is happening in the world; I don't want to isolate myself and become satisfied. I don't want to turn out like my parents, who are humanists—they care about people and all, but they don't believe in taking risks.

One analogy I make about my life is that it's like growing up as a white in Rhodesia ten years ago, being part of a small section of society which is really riding on the backs of the rest of the people. Now, I could go and be a GP in Salisbury and never deal with the awful hardships and basic oppression of the blacks, because it would be possible to ignore it. In the same way, doctors are not going to be the people changing this country, because they've got a vested interest not to. The change will come from the outside, from people putting the pinch on doctors. Medicine will always be a step behind other social change.

So this year I was struggling with what to do, trying to figure out what my potential role in life could be, given the skills that I have. I think the skills are valuable, and it would be stupid to throw them away. It happened that three different people started talking to me about the Mozambique government looking for doctors, since they had had a revolution. It caught me at a time where I wanted to work for somebody who I felt was doing the right thing, someplace where it would make a difference. The success or failure of a new Socialist country like Mozambique is going to have an incredible effect on the rest of Africa, the rest of the world. So that's where I'm going, to work as a resource person for other people who are making decisions. I'll still operate on some sort of social-policeman role, but at least I'll be doing it for the side I believe in!

Of course I'm not sure yet what position I'll play over there. I'm going openminded, knowing that I have a certain number of skills, which are useful in certain contexts. Poor people are really dying over there. But I'm going to try to use as much energy as I can to understand the situation. Even though I might be put in the role of foreign expert showing people how we do it in America, I want to turn it around and say, "Listen, you can do it just as well as I can, so don't rely on us, rely on yourselves." This may be hard, because many Africans, particularly in the cities, are very much attuned to Western medicine and look at it as an ultimate goal to strive for. It's hard to make judgments like this while I'm still in the U.S., but I think self-reliance is an important thing for everyone and Africans particularly, because colonialism has infringed on them over the last century, and I think one of the worst things I could do would be to take our system of medical care and impose it on those people, furthering the dependency and not even being appropriate.

I went into med school with a class that was coming out of college right at the height of unrest and demonstration in the sixties. Four years later I looked at the freshman medical-school class and couldn't believe how conservative they had become. This is also true among my friends. I've watched so many of them, one by one, stop trying quite so hard, begin to settle back into something more comfortable, to have kids, to lose their political sense or hope of changing the system. And that's been hard.

We Have to Change

BENJAMIN SPOCK, PEDIATRICIAN

"He certainly doesn't look like a doctor," cautioned matronly Mrs. Gary at the Rent-a-Car desk of the Fayetteville, Arkansas, airport. "I see him come through every few weeks; he's always off somewhere giving speeches. Most of the time he's with his wife. She sure doesn't look like a doctor's wife. Now, of course, mind you, I never used his book."

"Dr. Spock?" replied the middle-aged woman in the bank teller's cage in Rogers, Arkansas. "Sure, he comes in here sometimes. What a personality that man has. He's got unusual ideas, all right, but he stands up for them. And he sure seems younger than seventy-six. Why, he bounds in here like a youngster."

The soybean fields around Rogers stretched as far as they could this September afternoon before giving way to rolled-up Ozark foothills, to hickory and oak woods already radiant with autumn colors. Woodpeckers flew across the narrow road as it carved through red clay, leading out of town past pickup trucks and small, white, frame farmhouses, fields, pastures, and stream beds thick with dogwood and sumac. A mile past the point where the asphalt gave way to gravel was the turnoff to Dr. Spock's house.

It was a modern structure, set on a slope beside a lake still dotted with the gray ghosts of trees that had died when the valley was flooded for a recent dam project. At a small dock below the house, two rowing shells bobbed at their mooring, a sign that Spock still enjoyed the sport that had brought him and his teammates on the Yale crew the Olympic gold medal at the 1924 Paris Olympics.

A large brass plaque on the front door proclaimed "No Smoking": Spock had broken the habit almost twenty years ago. The door opened to the visitor's knock, and a tall, white-bearded man stood there smiling. Benjamin Spock's kindly greenish eyes sparkled behind the bifocals resting on his bulbous nose. He spoke in deep, reassuring tones, giving a tour of the house and proudly showing off the solar-heating panels and the porch outside the kitchen where squirrels panhandled daily. He moved as effortlessly as the woman in the bank had described.

Spock sat back down at the breakfast table with his wife Mary Morgan, an Arkansas native and a quick-witted advocate of such progressive causes as women's rights and vegetarianism. "It was really a matter of coming around to her point of view or starving to death," said Spock with a laugh, holding aloft a forkful of something that was definitely not meat.

His accent was southern New England blue-blooded, but redolent of humor and even traced with shyness. His voice came full-bodied from the broad chest, then suddenly turned to a whisper or a peep as he mimicked a child or mimicked himself.

In an era of medical sophistication, Dr. Spock wrote *Baby and Child Care*, which immediately after its publication in 1946 became the standard guide for parents on how to raise children. It has yet to be adequately replaced. Selling three-quarters of a million copies for many years and translated into every major language, *Baby and Child Care* effectively educated the lay public in the facts and methods of preventive medicine. "Trust yourself," it begins; "you know more than you think you do." It became a symbol of postwar living, and the children of the baby boom became the "Spock Generation."

It was in defense of this generation that Spock moved from his later teaching career at Western Reserve Medical School to the political sphere. In 1962 he became cochairman of SANE (National Committee for a Sane Nuclear Policy) and, in 1965 and later, became involved in activism against the war in Vietnam. For this he was indicted in 1968, tried, convicted, sentenced to two years in jail, but later acquitted, for conspiracy to aid and abet resistance to the draft. He was nominated for the presidency by the Peoples Party in 1972 and for the vice-presidency in 1976, thus becoming the most visible physician on the American political scene. In the later 1970s he worked against American reliance on nuclear power, which raised the hackles of the local Ku Klux Klan in Arkansas. He received several telephone threats but continued to receive mail at Box N (for "No Nukes") in Rogers.

As he sat in his living room, sharing thoughts about the Spock generation, particularly the ones who have now become medical students and young physicians, Spock didn't seem "controversial" for any of the usual reasons. He was not contentious, hard-driving, or rigidly dogmatic. Rather, his special qualities seemed to spring from a persistent, self-renewing youthfulness in the way he viewed his life and the world he had so deeply affected.

Practically all of us humans grew up in a family and were loved and cherished in one way or another, and this leads to the very strong impulse to try and do for others what was done to us and for us. This shows up very clearly in the three-, four-, or five-year-old girls and boys who play house all day long. "You be the mother, I'll be the father, and we'll use this other child or this doll for a baby. . . ." The father says, "Well, dear, it's time for me to go to work; is there anything you want me to bring home today?" And she says, "You might get me some eggs, and do take my car to the repair shop," or whatever she's heard her mother say. I remember watching a bossy four-and-a-half-year-old showing doll care to a mousey three-year-old. The four-and-a-half-year-old undressed the doll and bathed the doll and dried the doll and powdered and diapered it, all the time saying, "See, dear, see how I do it, dear?" Finally, after fifteen minutes, she said to the three-year-old, "Now you try it." The three-year-old stepped forward, and pretty soon the four-and-a-half-year-old said in a condescending tone, "No, dear, not like that, dear. . . . Now, watch me more carefully, dear." That older child had already become a parent in the spitting image of her mother. When she's twenty-four and a half she'll be talking to her true baby in the same sickly-sweet, condescending tones. [Laugh]

There's this *drive* to repeat the positive and the negative experiences of our childhood. You see children between three and six loving their dolls, yelling at their dolls, beating their dolls. The strongest impulse is to hurry and grow up in order to do for others what was done to you. At three, four, and five the desire is to get married and have children of your own, but after six years of age your horizon expands beyond that to the outside world. The identification with parents is especially strong for the first child, who on the average I think gets more pain from sibling rivalry than subsequent children do. One of the ways to assuage this rivalry is to pretend that you're not a child, to say scornfully to your mother when you're three years old and a new baby comes, "Look, Mama, look at the mess that he's making; look, he pooed all over the place." Statistics show that there's a preponderance of first children in the helping professions because, I think, they make such a strong early identification with their parents. I'm sure it was true in my case. I was the oldest of six children, and before long I was helping to give bottles and change diapers, and I suppose it's the most obvious reason why I went into pediatrics.

Of course, I missed the competitive premedical experience, because in the 1920s it was as easy as pie to get into medical school. I got into Yale Medical School with a C average. That enrages premedical students whom I talk to today. [Laughs] During my freshman year at college I just went over to the medical school and said, "In case I decide on medicine, what courses should I take?" They listed the chemistry, physics, and biology, and said, "We'll be glad to have you." It was great for a freshman to hear that from anyone.

As a C-average person, I am prejudiced against the heavy emphasis now placed on grades in getting into medical school today; I'm not sure that getting an A in chemistry has anything to do with being a good doctor. It is the laboratory faculties at medical schools that now determine who gets in. And what they select for is students who are easy for them to teach, who cope well with exams in the preclinical sciences.

In my college class, the social leaders expected to go into banking or brokerage. The idea was to make a million dollars by the age of forty or forty-five and then retire and play golf for the rest of one's life. And back then you couldn't get rich in medicine the way you could in banking or brokerage.

While I was still in college, someone gave me Cushing's *Life of William Osler* to read. Osler was a distinguished professor of medicine at Hopkins, and I became very depressed reading the biography. The author implied that there were three requirements to be a good doctor. One was that from early childhood one's predominant interest was science. Osler was always getting algae out of a pond under the guidance of a priest or someone who was a biologist and who would let him look at the algae through his microscope. But I had never been a boy-scientist. The second thing was that a doctor had no business marrying until he was a very successful person late in his career. That was true of Osler—he only married because he needed somebody to preside at the dinner table when he had distinguished guests from England and Germany. I knew I was going to get married—that I was very susceptible and couldn't possibly wait until I was distinguished. And the third thing about Osler was that he loved old people. Well, I still don't. [Laugh] My wife, Mary, has to remind me that I'm old myself. So this book about America's most prominent physician made me wonder whether I was going into the right field.

As an undergraduate I majored in English and minored in history but was compelled to take a course in either psychology or philosophy. I thought they were both goofy subjects, though I didn't know anything about either of them. Psychology seemed the lesser evil. The instructor was as dull as dishwater. Every day he drew a diagram of a neuron on the blackboard. Who cares about neurons at that age!

When I entered medical school I soon became depressed. I'd had a high old time as an undergraduate. But I found medical school *extremely* boring and oppressive: no more famous brilliant English teachers, no more Scroll and Key Society, no more eight-oared rowing victories (including the Olympics). All those things that I'd eaten up as an undergraduate were gone. All there was to do was study anatomy. I wanted to be a doctor but I didn't want to study the clavicle.

Throughout medical school there was almost no psychiatry taught. Yale didn't have psychiatrists on the faculty, so they invited a series of visiting lecturers to come and give talks. After two years at Yale I transferred to the College of Physicians and Surgeons at Columbia, and while they had some psychiatrists on the staff, all they did was to give us the table of classification of mental illness. There were the organic psychoses, and the inorganic psychoses, and then there were some psychoneuroses. That was all we got.

The first interest that I can remember in the psychological side of medicine was when I was a medical intern at Presbyterian Hospital in New York. Toward the end of this two-year service I was assigned to the private-patient service and had a middle-aged patient whose problem was that he had been slightly depressed almost all of his life. I didn't know how to put that on his medical record. I didn't want to chop up his history into those arbitrary divisions of family history, review of systems, personal history, present illness. So what I did was really bold. [Laughs] I wrote it all out as a story, including what his family was like and how he felt about his life.

Then I had a pediatrics residency for one year. Soon after I started that I began to feel that I had to get some kind of psychological training. I wrote to three pediatricians who were said to be interested in the psychological side, asking them where I could get some training. They all replied that there was no such training. So I settled for a year's adult psychiatric residency at New York Hospital. There I was just taking care of manic-depressive and schizophrenic patients, and this gave me no idea how to practice pediatrics. But I found that the psychoanalysts on the staff were the ones who make the cases interesting. So in 1933 I began both pediatric practice and a personal psychoanalysis. A year later I began taking two psychoanalytic seminars a week, which I kept up for five years.

Those first five years of practice were very painful because I was trying to reconcile psychoanalytic concepts with what mothers were telling me about their children. They didn't seem to fit at all. Only a few women in New York then wanted to breast feed, either because they'd been psychoanalyzed or they'd been reading psychology, or they were the wives of psychoanalysts, or perhaps they were psychiatric social workers. There was a disproportionate number of such women in my practice. But breast feeding was very difficult to arrange: private patients stayed in the hospital twelve days after delivery, and the babies couldn't be brought to the mother for the first twenty-four hours after delivery. When babies *were* brought in they came in exactly on a four-hour schedule. Babies couldn't be brought to their mother at two A.M. "The mother needs her rest," the obstetrician would say. There was nobody to encourage the mother or give her instruction about how to breast feed. The nurses in the nurseries at New York Hospital would say things to mothers like "You won't be able to breast feed with breasts like that!" Or "Your poor baby is crying with hunger all the time, what are you trying to prove?" The mother's female relatives were often deliberately discouraging.

This kind of disapproval that the mother got from almost everybody would break her down in a couple of days so that she'd be crying when I came in, and she'd say, "I don't want to breast feed!" I would get impatient and say, "You came to me because you wanted to breast feed your baby, and now's the time to stick with it." So the poor mother would be squeezed between me and the nursery staff. [Laugh]

At that time the rule in pediatrics was rigidity. Rigidity in feeding schedules, early toilet training, getting the baby off of the bottle and onto the cup. This wasn't because of overt hostility to babies [laugh]; it was just that pediatricians were anxious to prevent the still prevalent and lethal diarrheal diseases and believed that the survival of infants required carefully made formulas given on exact feeding schedules.

When an editor from Doubleday came to me after I'd been practicing five years and said, "Would you write a book for parents?" I said, "I don't know enough." That wasn't because I was modest. It was because I had not yet resolved the many seeming contradictions between psychoanalytic concepts and what mothers were telling me about their babies' and children's behavior.

Five years after *that* (ten years after starting practice), an editor of Pocket Books asked me to write a book. (The reason that publishers got to me was not because I was well known—I was unknown—but because I was the only pediatrician with psychiatric and psychoanalytic training.) The editor said jokingly that it didn't have to be a very good book because, at twenty-five cents a copy, they could sell 100,000 copies a year anyway. This was helpful to me, for if he had said they wanted it to be the best damned book ever written on the subject, that would have worried my perfectionism. Anyway I felt that I was ready because I now had answers for most of the troublesome questions that formerly baffled me, such as: Why do infants who are given a choice seem to prefer bottle to breast feeding? What is the explanation for the intense attachment of some young children to stuffed animals and blankets? Why do so many three- to five-year-olds have phobias, and should they all have therapy?

People ask how I thought I could write a book. All Spocks of my generation had to learn how to write because my tyrannical mother demanded of any child who was away from home two long letters a week, telling just what he'd done every morning, afternoon, and evening, who he did it with, and what kind of a person the friend was. She didn't want her children to be corrupted by unsuitable companions.

So I went about writing the manuscript fairly cautiously, rewriting it three times and making twenty-four copies and sending them to pediatricians and other specialists to criticize. My apartment was relatively small, and soon it was filled with enormous stacks of paper, just masses of stuff. Finally the publisher said, "Okay, we're going to press!" I fed all the drafts into the incinerator, it was such a relief. Later I found that such a manuscript would have been worth at least $50,000.

When it was published, most doctors felt that *Baby and Child Care* was a good book. They thought it helped them, and this surprised me, since I had anticipated criticism for telling mothers too much medical and psychological information—much of it newfangled, too.

(When I was on my way to the Paris Olympics in 1924, there was a very old-fashioned and successful doctor on the boat who took a fatherly interest in me because I was planning to go to medical school. I remember him telling me in a solemn manner, "Son, don't tell the patients anything. They won't understand. Just tell them not to worry, that you'll take care of everything. You have to keep control.")

So I was worried about the reaction of the medical profession, and I remember anxiously waiting for the review in the *Journal of the American Medical Association*. The review said that it was a pretty good book. The only criticism was that it too often said, "Consult your own physician." [Laugh] I just loved reading that.

Even today, the only thing about the book that irritates pediatricians is to have mothers say, "That's not what Spock says." I mentioned that once in a talk to the Academy of Pediatrics, and there was such a roar of laughter from the audience that it nearly blew the windows out.

There is still a gulf between pediatrics and psychology, and in most pediatric services. You feel this as the pediatrician on the staff, who is trying to teach the emotional side of pediatrics. Such pediatricians are apt to feel abused or at least unappreciated, and they're always getting together at conferences to console each other. One of the lamentations you hear is that when certain individuals, who were really interested in the emotions as medical students, get into their pediatric residency training, they sometimes act ashamed of ever having known the psychological-minded pediatrician or child psychiatrist. They avoid his glance when they meet him going down the hall. It's what you call in child psychiatry "loyalty conflict." During their residency they're identifying with the chief of pediatrics, who is usually a scientist and who often has no real sympathy for the psychological side, even though he may think it would be good to have one captive psychological-minded pediatrician on his staff for the sake of appearance!

The residency is where you're getting ready to go out and become some kind of doctor, and this intensifies the need to watch every move of the head of the service, to identify with him, mimic his actions and interests. This leads to a great deal of disappointment for many of the residents who go into pediatrics practice, since of course what they're learning is the diagnosis and treatment of the rare condition, and they've been misled into thinking that pediatrics practice consists of making difficult diagnoses. They soon find out that practice means dribbly noses and formulas and anxious parents. You hear one practitioner say to another [whispers], "At last I've got an interesting case. I want you to feel the tip of the spleen." [Laughs] If you want to be an interesting patient, the first requirement is to have an enlarged spleen. That makes doctors' eyes sparkle.

I think that the reason that a great majority of professors of pediatrics have always been uncomfortable with the psychological—and the same goes for professors of medicine—is that they are basically hired for their scientific ability and they tend to be afraid of their own feelings—other people's and their own. One of the things that you can do when you're afraid of your feelings is to intellectualize, to view everything around you in impersonal, abstract terms. Of course, if a physician broke down and wept every time a patient was in danger of dying, he'd be a very unsatisfactory doctor. There has to be a compromise between retaining your sensitivity for the feelings of the patient and yet preserving enough professional detachment. It's the uncommon person who can remain a good scientist and be really empathetic about feelings. This is too bad, but it has to be faced. Intellectuality can be a defense against feeling, and medical students should be taught this so that they can be on guard to some degree.

I think Abraham Flexner made a mistake in his report of 1910 in concluding that one should have at least three years of undergraduate arts and science *before* going to medical school. I think that what they ought to have done was integrate a broad variety of premedical subjects into a six-year medical course. It's wrong for the students entering medical school to feel that they are "finished" with English, or that they've already "taken" anthropology. [Laughs] The time to study anthropology and sociology is while you're learning about and having experiences with patients. And teachers of English should keep you from acquiring the hackneyed language of medicine.

At Case Western Reserve Medical School, where I taught for

twelve years, the curriculum involves assigning to each first-year student a family to be responsible for. The student functions somewhat as that family's primary-care physician, though the responsibility scares the be jeebers out of them, such experience is valuable in order to counteract the depersonalization that happens in most schools. For example, our students would become indignant when they heard that their pregnant patient, had been treated rudely in the clinic, or called by her first name by a callous obstetrical resident. They would come in to a preceptor session quivering with indignation about this humiliation of their patient. I used to answer, "I'm sorry, but you can't change the hospital system right now. What you can do is to keep yourself from becoming callous when *you* are a resident."

Of course, I feel that this sort of direct experience should not be confined to medical school. I think people preparing for the ministry or for the law should be dealing with people continuously, and discussing the emotional aspects of their experiences. For I'm sure that many ministers of the gospel aren't comforting at all, and I know from personal experience that many lawyers are impossible to understand.

The first-year students at Case Western Reserve would be embarrassed when their patient families called them "Doctor," because the students knew they were four years away from being doctors. They would remind their patients of this. Then the students would fall into traps like picking up the mother and driving her to the clinic for her checkup because otherwise she would have to take two buses. Or they would lend the family money. These were nice impulses but you confuse the professional role if you also become a taxi driver or money lender. I used to say to students, "*After* you become a doctor and are sure of your own identity you can relax in any direction you want, but when you're trying to find out what your relationship is to patients you ought to be a little bit cautious."

In retrospect I am glad to have taken all those fascinating English and history courses at Yale. I think that the college years should be a time for the fullest savoring of other fields aside from the one you plan to enter. It broadens perspective.

I got into opposition of the war in Vietnam without meaning to. I joined SANE in 1962 because I was persuaded that if we didn't get a test-ban treaty, more and more children around the world would be born with mental and physical defects and would die of cancer. But SANE had to approach me three times before the message finally got under my skin.

In the 1964 election I was asked to publicly support Johnson because he said he would not send Americans to fight in Asia. When he did, I became deeply involved in protesting the war. And that experience radicalized me. For the young people in college, the motivating factor was being threatened with the draft, with having to go and kill and be killed in a faraway place where these young people knew our country had no business whatsoever, in a war that was completely ignoble. They became highly critical not only of American foreign policy, but of their universities, of archaic parietal rules and the suppression of free speech, as well as the mistreatment of minorities and women.

Between 1965 and 1973, I was on the road half the weeks of the year, speaking at six universities a week, five appearances a day. But I was always impressed with how little activism there was in medical schools compared with undergraduate colleges. It was very, very rare for me to be asked to speak at a medical school.

I thought that young people's whole attitude toward life had changed for the better in the late sixties and early seventies. I was inspired by their idea of moving from a competitive to a cooperative society, and of seeing how simply one could live instead of how ostentatiously. To me those were startling new ideas, and I was converted to them. I not only hoped but expected that this trend would go on.

At this time; people like Reverend Norman Vincent Peale, Jr., and Spiro Agnew started blaming me for the "permissive" upbringing of youth. The accusation that I corrupted a whole generation is ridiculous. I was never accused of being permissive until I was indicted by the federal government for conspiracy in 1968, and all the accusations came from people who were supporting the war and who had never used my book. A typical hate letter would say, "Thank God I never used your horrible book. That's why my children take baths and study in school." [Laugh] Of course even the students who were conservative and were willing to be drafted were also raised on my book. (It was selling three-quarters of a million copies each year.) On the other hand, I still get stopped by people who recognize me on the street and in airports, and they'll say in a really friendly and loving voice, "You've helped me so much to raise two fine children." And often they'll add, "I don't see that your book is permissive." [Laugh] It isn't permissive at all. It says to respect your children, but also to ask your children to respect you; ask for cooperation, politeness, and give them firm leadership. I have a clear conscience about that. I never told parents to let their children have anything, do anything they want.

But while I was not a wholesale corrupter of youth, I do think it's possible that I contributed to the different attitudes that young people developed in the 1960s. I'm thinking particularly of the self-assurance of young people, of their relative insensitivity to adult disapproval. Two years before I had to retire at Western Reserve, I was responsible for the first-year series of lecture course in clinical science. I recruited the speakers and gave about a quarter of the lectures myself. Within a month after medical school started, a third of the first-year students would come late to class, and also bring coffee in paper cups to drink during lectures. At first they would just take surreptitious sips and then put the cups down, but after a while they got bolder, and they could hold a cup to their lips all through the lecture. I could see their eyes looking scornfully at me over the rim of their cups as if they were saying, "What crap!"

I said to the class that they didn't have to come, but that if they did come they should arrive on time and without coffee. It didn't make the slightest impression. So the next time I decided to let my indignation and irritation show, so I thundered a little. It was enough to make gooseflesh go up and down my own spine to hear me shouting in the austere amphitheater. This didn't make the least difference either. I tried stony silence. If I was lecturing and someone came in late I'd stop right in the middle of a sentence, sternly watching this person climb up to a seat, and imagining her or him red in the face and ducking into the first seat. Not at all. She'd saunter up, wave to friends, and then turn around smiling as if to say, "You may proceed, any time."

When I was in medical school, we were afraid of the faculty, and if a lowly instructor scowled with one eyebrow, students would whisper to one another, "What was Brown angry about?" We had an acute sensitivity to disapproval. It has vanished among today's youth.

The worst of it came that January, when the class sent an official committee to complain that the course I was so proud of and that previous classes had loved had no content, that it was just fluff. I was afraid that the dean and the rest of the faculty would hear about this, since a majority of the faculty disapproved of teaching clinical science in the first year, and they only allowed this course because the students were eager to play doctor. So, I had tried to intimidate the students, but they ended up by intimidating me.

My theory is that it isn't rudeness, it's a lack of antennae for disapproval. And this is because in early childhood, these individuals weren't intimidated by their parents. Their parents believed Freud and Dewey and Spock when they said that "children aren't born evil." The message to parents was that "if you love them and ask for respect from them and give them guidance (because they're inexperienced and impulsive), you'll find that they *want* to grow up. You don't have to force growing up on them, you don't have to be on guard all the time!" In other words, if they weren't intimidated in childhood it's too late to try to intimidate them in medical school." [Laugh]

Many years ago, some significant experiments were performed to determine the difference in effect of autocratic and democratic discipline. Boys about ten to fourteen years old were assigned to after-school-activity clubs with psychologists playing the role of either a democratic or an autocratic group leader. The autocratic leader would say, in effect, to his group, "Okay, we're going to have this club for the next ten weeks. I want you to pay attention to business. I'll tell you what we're going to do. We're going to make birdhouses. If you don't behave, you'll have to leave the club."

The democratic leader tells his group, "Kids, this is your club.

You can decide what we are going to do with it. Are we going to study nature or make something or read stories?"

There was also a "laissez-faire" group with a leader who didn't say anything at all. He was just around in case anybody wanted to speak with him. His group was chaos. [Laughs]

To make it scientific, each leader took turns playing the different roles, and each group of kids got to experience the three different types of discipline. Well, they found that the autocratic leadership got the birdhouses built with the least fuss and delay. The democratic group took at least twice as long. But when the democratic leader went out of the room, the work went on almost as efficiently as when the leader was in the room, whereas when the autocrat left his group alone, the kids would find the most defenseless group member and tease and beat up on him, taking out their pent-up hostility.

The researchers also found that the kids made a relatively easy transition from the democratic group to the autocratic, even though there would be some grousing. Soon, the kids would knuckle under and do what they were told. The most difficult and painful transition for them to make was from the autocratic to the democratic group, since to be let free after being bossed around made all the restlessness and hostility come busting out.

When I was at Yale Medical School, we were allowed to study as we wished, and we didn't have to take any examinations for two years. I was unable to benefit from this sudden freedom. I slacked off and did nothing. I couldn't make myself work. Part of the reason was that all the way through my schooling, whatever natural curiosity and enthusiasm I had about learning was gradually squelched, and I was always made to feel that I had to study because the teacher (backed up by my parents) said so.

My ideal would be a philosophy of education from nursery school on through to the end of medical school in which natural desire to learn is the motivating force. Obviously that's what you have to rely on after you get out of medical school.

A study of practicing doctors concluded that there was absolutely no correlation between a doctor's medical-school class rank and how competent and conscientious a doctor he or she was a dozen years later. The people who were practicing superior medicine and the people who were practicing inferior medicine came equally from the three thirds of their medical-school classes. That is the most disconcerting study I've ever heard of—it's nihilistic. It almost means that it doesn't matter whether you go to medical school at all. The important thing is what motivates you after you get out on your own. It certainly means that we are justified in experimenting as widely and as wildly as we wish with medical education, for we have no idea what makes a doctor good ten years later.

If you want to know how medicine is going to change—you have to know how the whole society is going to change. Some people say that human nature is fixed, but I believe that ideals are constantly changing and sometimes changing drastically. I'm asked to talk to high-school students here in Rogers, and I've found them interested in hearing about socialism (to which I was converted by my opposition to the war in Vietnam), and about the dangers of nuclear power and nuclear weapons. At the high-school age many of them still have open minds and are not intensely materialistic. But I think that as they get closer and closer to choosing an occupation, a profession, the attitudes of the teacher they identify with become very powerful, whether the model is maternalistic or idealistic, interested in the rare disease or in common problems.

I believe that we will have a destruction of the world from nuclear weapons unless a change in the whole political and economic system intervenes, or unless we get a relatively minor disaster such as a million people being killed in some nuclear-weapons disaster, enough to scare the hell out of everybody, so that there is a worldwide demand to eliminate such weapons.

If we're going to survive, we have to change, and one of the problems with changing a technological society is that the people in technology tend to have blinders on. Medicine is a collection of technologies, and that's why so many people in medicine have so little insight into what is going on in the outside world.

The telephone had rung. A man from a radio station in Columbia, Mississippi, was on the line, hoping for a fifteen-minute interview.

Spock picked up the receiver beside the couch and after listening for a moment, began to speak. "What do I think of today's youth? I like the young people of today. They have ideals; they make their own decisions much more than we did as kids. Am I going to write any more books? No! I'm seventy-six and I've written ten, and that's plenty."

His words carried out over the still surface of the lake. His wife had spoken of how special, how rare it had been to take a picnic to an island in the lake the previous day, when they both put all of their responsibilities aside and spent hours sunbathing and swimming. The world had followed Benjamin Spock even to this Ozark hideaway, because it knew he had something to say.

Conclusion

I had a friend in college who wanted very much to go to medical school. A year older than I, he was filled with a genuine warmth for the people around him. A student of classical music, he gave recitals of his own compositions on the bassoon. Sometimes after dinner he would get out his accordion and organize impromptu square dances on the lawn outside the college dining hall.

We took organic chemistry together. The course had a reputation for bringing out the ruthless, competitive nature in premedical students. But this friend transcended that atmosphere. He laughed aloud and even sang during laboratory, sharing his equipment and his always excellent results.

During his senior year, the rejection letters from medical schools began to arrive. Each week it seemed a little harder for him to smile and shrug off the bad news. When he stood on the lawn playing madrigals and reels, he hit the notes with new determination and intensity. When the last rejection letter came, he signed up to take the Medical College Admissions Test once again. Before the test he talked with me, full of plans for reapplying, of one day becoming a physician.

The MCAT lasted from eight in the morning until six at night. The educators who create such tests had recently revised it. They had eliminated the general-knowledge section and made the rest of the test longer and more science oriented.

One hundred of us sat in the stiff seats, penciling in innumerable blanks on computer sheets. We consumed cookies, soft drinks, anything to stay alert. Hours dragged by. There was none of the intense sprinting of a final examination. This was a marathon.

During the lunch break, I sprawled on a grassy hill, gulping fresh air. Out of the corner of my eye, I saw my red-haired friend walking away. He never returned for the afternoon portion of the test.

"I was halfway through the physics section," he told me later, "when I reached my limit. For years I had been trying and trying to get into medical school, to be a doctor, and all at once there was nothing left inside of me to keep trying. I just didn't want to compete against all those people anymore. If medical school is anything like the MCAT, it's not right for me anyway."

I think of him sometimes when I am studying late at the medical school, the desks around me occupied by other medical students and the atmosphere reminiscent of the MCAT. When I last heard of him, he was playing folk music in the Berkshire Hills of New England. In my thoughts he is happy, at peace with himself and his decision. But what has medicine lost by turning him away? The profession turned away a generous human being who had a sure grasp of science but who cared more about people.

All is not well with the medical profession. The recognition of this runs through the words of the doctors in this book. Something is wrong and the symptoms are widespread: alcoholic and drug-addicted physicians, dissatisfied patients, and escalating costs.

Doctors like William Foege have learned that preventing disease is more effective than trying to cure symptoms. It is time to apply that lesson to the medical profession itself. Its problems seem to stem directly from the attitudes of individual physicians and the expectations of their patients. How can these problems be solved?

The young people who satisfy medical-school admissions committees enter those medical schools as individuals. Like the medical students and physicians in this book, they change during the years that follow. Does a rigid system of education mold their personalities into a professional stereotype? Certainly such an established and powerful institution of medical schools and training programs is a force to reckon with in this regard. But I believe that the strongest determinants of physicians' attitudes are the personal qualities students possess when they begin medical school.

If medicine is to solve some of its own problems, medical schools need to select a different breed of student. It has not been enough to select and train doctors according to the scientific guidelines that Flexner proposed almost seventy years ago. There is a need for doctors who can use science and technology as tools while recognizing the limitations of such tools in their dealings with individual patients.

Medicine also needs a new breed of patients. The consumer movement in this country has made strides to demand better health care, to demystify medical procedures, to protest high medical fees. But this movement cannot afford to stop there. Patients must become informed partners in the healing process, rather than the adversaries of physicians, and some of these informed consumers should consider entering medical school themselves.

Medicine needs more people like Dr. David Gomez who have an instinctive human touch and are not left insensitive by the conditioning of medical education and training. Medicine needs more people like Ellen Salzman who bring unique and vital perspectives to their work. It needs people who can talk and listen to patients not fluent in the technical language of medicine. It needs more people willing to place service to others above personal gain. Yet many of these people, like my musical friend, become discouraged during the premedical years or before.

As Tim Morton found out, medical-school admissions committees have become more conservative in recent years. They are more intent than ever on following quantitative, objective criteria, such as MCAT scores, in their decisions. After the expansion years of the 1960s and 1970s, medical schools are again reducing their class sizes in response to fears of a forthcoming "doctor glut." Federal-loan programs for medical students are declining, for the same reason. Gradually, the people entering medical school are coming from a smaller and wealthier segment of society. The doors of the medical profession are closing on the people whom medicine needs most. This book is a call to those people. It is time to open those doors wider than ever.